The Enzyme Advantage
FOR WOMEN

Also by Dr. Howard F. Loomis, Jr.

Enzymes: The Key to Health, Volume 1, The Fundamentals

The Enzyme Advantage: For Health Care Providers and People Who Care About Their Health

The Enzyme Advantage

FOR WOMEN

HOWARD F. LOOMIS, JR., D.C., F.I.A.C.A.

WITH ARNOLD MANN

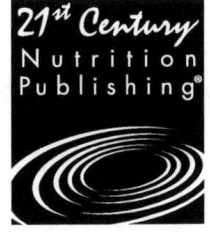

Copyright © 2016 by Dr. Howard Loomis, Jr.
Published by 21st Century Nutrition Publishing®
800-662-2630

Without limiting the rights under copyright reserved above, no part of this publication may be reproduced, stored in, or introduced into a retrieval system, or transmitted, in any form or by any means (electronic, mechanical, photocopying, recording, or otherwise), without the prior written permission of both the copyright owner and the above publisher of this book, except for brief excerpts or quotations in a book review.

Cover design, layout: Camron Lewis
Editor: Meredith H. Pond

Library of Congress Cataloging-in-Publication Data
Loomis, Howard F.
The Enzyme Advantage for Women
Includes references and index.
1. Enzymes. 2. Nutrition. 3. Digestion. 4. Chiropractic.
Mann, Arnold.

First Edition, Printed in the USA

ISBN 978-0-9769124-2-2

DISCLAIMER: This book is not about treating disease, and no information contained in it should be construed as such. This book is about how plant enzymes can be used to deliver nutrition, for the purpose of restoring normal function and maintaining health. When making dietary changes, please remember to consult your health care practitioner.

Acknowledgments

Without the help of highly educated, professional and dedicated women, I could not have completely developed the much needed material for this book.

I am grateful to have had, for many years, the capable assistance of **Cheryl Rupard** as my executive assistant whose guidance has been invaluable. Among many other things, she has taught me to be patient and calm, and not to jump to conclusions.

Polly Fleming came to me immediately after college and manages my lecturing schedule and appointments and has many projects that would otherwise escape my attention. Among other things, she has taught me to be "redundant" when necessary in my writings and lectures.

Last, but certainly not least, is *Laura Anne Sawall* my researcher and in-house editor who makes certain I stay on time and on track with my articles and books.

I am sure you will recognize as you read this book the many contributions they made and helped me to understand.

Dedication

Without help there is no way I could have understood the complexities women are confronted with in their daily lives concerning menstruation and reproduction.

I have the education to understand the physiological and nutritional implications of the problems. But without guidance, so necessary in a young man's life, to appreciate the role of women in our society, my life's journey would have been quite different.

Don't look for anything chauvinistic here, my mother and both grandmothers never stood for it – from their husbands or me.

It is to:

**Clara Elizabeth Budde,
Mary Ellen Barnett, and
Catherine Marie Coughlin
that this book is lovingly dedicated.**

TABLE OF CONTENTS

FOREWORD—BY DR. ANN MILLER 1

INTRODUCTION—BY DR. HOWARD LOOMIS, JR. 5

CHAPTER 1
    Cracking the Code: *The Difference Proper Nutrition Makes* . . . 11

CHAPTER 2
    In the Beginning: *From Childhood to Puberty* 43

CHAPTER 3
    What Could Go Wrong? *The Young Adult Years* 63

CHAPTER 4
    A Balancing Act: *From Prevention to Pregnancy* 91

CHAPTER 5
    And So It Begins: *The Perimenaupausal Years* 121

CHAPTER 6
    It's Not Over: *Menaupause and Beyond* 145

Epilogue: *The Final Word* 159

GLOSSARY 163

SELECTED BIBLIOGRAPHY 177

INDEX 181

ABOUT THE AUTHORS 189

Foreword
By Dr. Ann Miller

As a health care provider, it has been my experience that women tend to wait before seeking help for their female health problems. These include things like loss of libido, changes in their menstrual cycle, bloating, cramping, the emotional upheavals—all the things that we are told are just a normal part of our monthly rhythm. They don't seek care until it becomes emotionally distressful for them. Because it's "normal." It's what it means to be female.

This thinking has been passed down through generations. The medical model offers little help to these patients, because it's basically exchanging one symptom for another. So while their menstrual cramps might improve, now they don't have any energy. By the time they got to me, they'd tried everything.

Before I was introduced to Dr. Loomis' work, I had a large nutritional component within my practice. I had some degree of success with various vitamins, minerals and thyroid supplements, along with supplements targeted at improving pituitary and uterine health. But I was never able to realize the consistent, reproducible success you want to see in your patients. A woman might feel better for a month or two, then she wouldn't feel better. So I couldn't stay with the same protocol. It seemed like the problem kept changing. I never felt I was getting to the source of the problem.

Then I got sick.

It started in 2007. I began having severe anxiety and panic attacks. I also had terrible menstrual cramps, I was constipated all the time, and I wasn't sleeping. I had little interest in cleaning or maintaining my home. The joy of motherhood—I had two small children at the time—had become work. I was barely able to maintain my practice of 20 years.

I don't tolerate medications very well, so the more they medicated me, the less I wanted to do—the less I lived my life. There were days when I couldn't make it to the grocery store without having to turn around and come home. I simply couldn't put myself in a public situation.

I tried psychotherapy, I tried acupuncture, I tried applied kinesiology with all its nutrition, I tried chiropractic, and I tried all the drugs from the medical community. Nothing helped. I would have a lessening of symptoms and feel pretty good for a while. Then, I would go to a concert with my husband, have a full blown panic attack and beg him to call me an ambulance.

After months of struggling, I met a practitioner who used the Loomis System®. After my labs were analyzed, I started taking the plant enzymes that best suited my symptoms and my lab results—designed to help me digest proteins. I have since had a complete and lasting resolution of my anxiety and panic attacks.

Looking back, I have always suffered from protein deficiency, and the calcium deficiency that accompanies it, as described in this book.

I started menstruating at age 10, and had a very heavy flow every month. It would exhaust me. I would have terrible cramps and wind up staying home from school. I probably had depression back then as well. I always had weight issues. All of my siblings were thin; I was the heavy one.

And, I noticed at a young age, whenever I ate a diet high in protein, I felt better. When I became sick and started seeing a psychologist, I remember saying to him that I was going to go back to the bodybuilding diet I was on during my 30's, because that was when I felt the best. Of course that was a high protein diet.

The Loomis System® made sense. I took the training and became a Loomis practitioner.

Now, I love coming to work. This system, combined with the chiropractic, brings everything together. Finally, all the physiology and biochemistry I learned during my chiropractic training made sense. What Dr. Loomis has put together is an integrative approach, recognizing that everything—the musculoskeletal system, the body's organ systems and the nervous system—are all connected. The key to restoring health is providing the right nutrition to the struggling systems to restore normal function.

And plant enzymes are the key.

It makes a lot of sense to look at the three main nutrients—protein, carbohydrates and fats—and determine where the patient is deficient. If you can pin that down, the rest will fall into place.

And it does. When my patients come back in a couple of weeks they are astounded. They're better rested and more alive. They feel more like themselves. They are more that person they want to be. They have more energy and they feel better overall, and their tolerance for their children has increased.

It affects everyone. Like they say, "When mom is happy, everybody's happy."

Because of Dr. Loomis' work with plant enzymes, I have been able to provide the many women coming to my office with hope.

As a woman and as a healer, it has been a privilege and an honor to learn from one of the best.

Introduction

The idea of writing this book first came to me in the fall of 2015, at a state of Wisconsin chiropractic conference where I was a featured speaker.

There were three of us speaking that morning. Each of our rooms were prepared to accommodate our expected share of the 200 attendees at this continuing education conference. We were all speaking on topics relative to chiropractic. I was speaking on women's health.

When I entered my room, about 60 of the chairs were taken. I had divided my allotted four hours into three sessions, with two 15-minute breaks in between. After the first break, I noticed more people coming in. Suddenly all the chairs were full! It soon became obvious that people were coming in from the other lectures. By the third session, the room was packed. People were standing all along the conference room walls.

I had a similar experience in the spring of 2015, in St. Louis. What was going on? That's what I was asking myself. What were the other speakers talking about? And, more importantly, why were people losing interest, or getting bored and coming in here?

It wasn't until afterwards that I realized there was a tremendous interest in women's health.

For me, I first became interested in women's health in 1980. I found that many of the life-disrupting symptoms associated with the ups and downs of my female patients' reproductive lives could be relieved by taking a nutritional approach—combining dietary modification with plant enzyme formulas designed to deliver specific nutrients to struggling organ systems, thus restoring normal function.

And it worked. My patients reported that they experienced an obvious change in symptoms with overall improvement. Before long I found myself writing on the subject, and lecturing too.

Back in 2003, I was giving a 12-hour lecture on the use of plant enzymes for health care professionals in Albuquerque, New Mexico, when two nurses invited me to breakfast and asked me to write about the use of supplemental plant enzymes for enhanced digestion in pregnancy.

At first I was somewhat dismissive of their idea. Each woman is unique, and what each woman needs is also unique based on a thorough examination and lab work and more.

"You're probably more qualified to write on that subject than I am," I said to them.

They assured me, however, they were not, and that they felt I could bring some clarity to the use of nutritional supplementation during pregnancy.

But what was I going to write about that hadn't already been written?

After months of contemplation I remembered a conversation I had with my mother. My mother and paternal grandmother were both nurses. I remembered them telling me that when a man and a woman get married, they should both prepare their bodies before they decide to have children.

Because of this remembered conversation, I decided that my first publication on women's health would be called: "The Five Stages of Pregnancy," beginning with both parents preparing themselves nutritionally before conception, with the future baby's health in mind, and then continuing through the first, second and third trimesters, to the months after delivery with both the baby's and the mother's postpartum health in mind.

Those were the five stages pregnancy, from preconception to postpartum stages.

All of this information appears in Chapter 4 of this book.

Seven years later, in 2010, after multiple requests for more information, I revisited that article in a 12-hour presentation on women's health issues for a conference I conduct annually. I had been doing these conferences for a professional audience since 2001, presenting a different topic every year. This was by far the most difficult and complex subject I had ever encountered.

In the year I spent researching the subject, I was struck by the struggle that many women have with "female" health issues throughout their lives — primarily by the enormous amount of conflicting information that is presented to them regarding how their bodies function and what they should do for this, that, or the other symptom to prevent the onset of a pathological process.

I wound up getting through the material, the presentation was well received, and it left a lasting impression on me.

The aha! moments kept coming, one at a time, *slowly*.

In the spring of 2015 I was asked to speak in St. Louis. My most lasting memory of that conference will always be that of a middle-aged physician who approached me on a break. She had brought her mother, who was spending time elsewhere in the hotel during the conference. The doctor was so excited about the material I was presenting that she asked if her mother could join the audience for the remainder of my presentation. I will never forget that conversation.

The idea that women need accurate, science-based information for maintaining their health was undeniable. However, the full importance of what I was getting into—the Big Picture, if you will—didn't really hit me until that morning at the 2015 Wisconsin conference when my presentation room began to fill with more and more male practitioners. Was it that they were going through what I went through in my own practice?

For me, it wasn't just the attentive audience, enduring standing room only, that got me. It was their eyes.

The audience that morning was a fairly equal distribution of male and female chiropractic practitioners. Due to a childhood hearing impairment, I have always paid close attention to people's eyes. Looking at the intent eyes in this audience this morning, I could see that they were all very interested in what I was saying. They stayed right with me. But when I hit on the topic of the Pill, everything changed.

Birth control pills are all designed to interfere with normal reproductive function. And these medicines all work differently, as we will see in Chapter 4 of this book. What it comes down to is that each woman has to find the pill that she is willing to tolerate regarding the side effects and accompanying symptoms in order to prevent pregnancy. It's all hit and miss. There is no definitive approach—women are individuals.

INTRODUCTION

When I started talking about the Pill, that's when the women's eyes in the audience changed. They lit up. Suddenly they went from, "Oh, that's interesting" to "Somebody finally understands!"

Women were coming up to me on break, saying, "This is wonderful. Could you do more of these talks?"

One man came up to me on a break. He was a chiropractor with a very active practice who was looking to retire. He had three recent graduates working in his office. They were all women, fresh out of school.

"They really need this," he told me. "Is there something you can do for them?"

I told him we had done seminars in Wisconsin about women's health, and we would be doing more.

That was the question that kept coming. "Would you present more on this subject at another time?"

But it was the eyes that really did it to me. An wave of possibility and awareness catching fire in each bright, intelligent mind.

And so this book.

— Dr. Howard F. Loomis, Jr.
Madison, Wisconsin, April 2016

CHAPTER 1

Cracking the Code

The Difference Proper Nutrition Makes

I had seen women suffering from premenstrual syndrome (PMS) before—hundreds of them in the 12 years since I opened my practice in May 1968. These women were desperate and looking for help, but there was little I or anyone else could do to give them relief from the vast array of symptoms identified with this disorder. If I were one of the local medical doctors, I could write a prescription to treat a bout with depression.

But when five women showed up at my door during a two-week period in October of 1980, each plagued by lifelong PMS symptoms, I had reason to believe that I might be able to help because I found a common diagnostic thread in each woman that opened the door of understanding for me.

For the first time, I had something that was going to give me the upper hand with PMS—this notoriously vexing and unrelenting adversary—if I could just figure out how to use it. If I could just crack the code.

Imagined?

Not long ago, PMS was seen as an "imagined" disease. Women reporting its symptoms were often told PMS was "all in their head." The first formal medical description of premenstrual syndrome goes back to a paper presented by Robert T. Frank in 1931 at the New York Academy of Medicine, and titled, "Hormonal Causes of Premenstrual Tension." The actual term *premenstrual syndrome* first appeared in an article in the *British Medical Journal* in 1953. Legitimization and definition of PMS as a medical condition has been an ongoing process; furthermore, the search for effective treatments has been disappointing at best.

Understanding PMS

To understand premenstrual syndrome, one must understand the dynamic relationship of estrogen and progesterone. For the sake of clarity, the first day of bleeding is used to mark the start of a cycle. The next cycle begins when bleeding again commences.

> Let's assume a 28-day cycle for description purposes. During that cycle, it is the fluctuating relationship between estrogen and progesterone that drives the emotional roller coaster related to menstruation. Normally for a woman's central nervous system, estrogen functions as a stimulant, and progesterone functions as a depressant.

About a week prior to ovulation, estrogen secretion increases and stimulates the maturation of the follicle. Ovulation occurs when the ovaries release an egg or ovum. This marks the beginning of the **luteal phase** of the menstrual cycle. Estrogen secretion now begins to drop, and progesterone secretion begins to increase slowly as the lining of a woman's uterus becomes thicker to prepare for a possible pregnancy. If pregnancy does not occur, both estrogen and progesterone secretion drop and the collection of symptoms known as premenstrual syndrome begins—until bleeding marks the onset of the next period.

Most women experience some cyclical bodily changes during their menstrual years, corresponding to this pattern of cycling hormones. Most of these changes are normal. Many ancient cultures observed and even ritualized these subtle shifts in body response, and mental and emotional focus. Some women express a positive attitude about the conscious observance of these patterns within their own bodies.

However, when the hormonal and chemical changes cause debilitating symptoms, they can disrupt the function of virtually all body systems, as well as a woman's emotional life.

What Are the Possible Symptoms?

Behavioral symptoms appear in the form of nervousness, irritability, agitation, unreasonable temper, fatigue and depression. Symptoms suggesting clinical depression—such as anxiety, palpitations, tightening in the chest, and hyperventilation—are common.

Neurological symptoms include headaches, vertigo (dizziness), syncope (temporary loss of consciousness due to a drop in blood pressure), paresthesia (tingling, prickling sensations) of the hands or feet, and aggravation of seizure disorders.

Gastrointestinal symptoms include constipation, increase or decrease in appetite, and carbohydrate cravings, particularly for sugar and chocolate.

Respiratory issues arise when asthma is intensified due to increased simple sugar consumption.

Other symptoms include edema (excess fluids collecting in body tissues), weight gain, backache, breast changes, joint and muscle pain, abdominal cramps, enuresis (involuntary urination), oliguria (production of abnormally small amounts of urine), capillary fragility, eye complaints, and exacerbations of dermatologic disease (e.g., acne).

By the Numbers

Breaking the data down demographically:

1. Eighty percent of women with PMS experience anxiety-related symptoms associated with excess estrogen as well as central nervous system stimulation resulting in feelings of anxiety.

2. Sixty percent of women with PMS experience bloating and edema.

3. Forty percent of women with PMS are overwhelmed by carbohydrate cravings due to increased energy demands and lack of adequate hormonal secretions, which usually involve poor lipid ingestion/digestion.

4. Only about 5 percent of PMS sufferers are primarily affected by depression related to excess progesterone, which causes central nervous system depression.

There is no part of the female body that PMS does not touch. Symptoms and intensity vary from woman to woman and from cycle to cycle.

At least 85 percent of menstruating women have at least one PMS symptom as part of their monthly cycle, while 3 to 8 percent have a more severe debilitating form of PMS called premenstrual dysphoric disorder (PMDD). A hotly debated condition, the existence of PMDD is denied by many experts.

Is it safe to say that any woman alive would give up her monthly period if she could get pregnant and bear her children another way? It's a fair question to ask.

If only science could get to the core of the problem—find some commonality—so we could open the door to an effective PMS treatment for all women.

Nutrition vs. Pharmacology

Back in the 1970s, a Columbia University study set out to find any commonality of PMS symptoms and came up with nothing. The study looked at 200 patients over a three-year period and found some 130 symptoms. The authors ultimately decided that PMS just didn't make any sense at all.

Their conclusion: PMS was not a treatable condition.

A more recent study documented more than 200 different symptoms associated with PMS.

Medical treatments for PMS today are mostly aimed at symptoms. Those include antidepressants, anti-inflammatory drugs for pain, and diuretics for water retention. Another "treatment," birth control pills, cause PMS symptoms in some women and reduce physical symptoms in others.

If there were only a way to get to the physiological cause, to break the code, so to speak. That's what I was trying to do back in the early years of my practice.

Is This Normal? No!

I never bought into the theory that PMS suffering is a normal process that comes with the menstrual cycle. For me, the symptoms plaguing women were due to an incomplete cycle, one not being completed normally. If the hormonal shifts occur normally, with proper balance, there should be no symptoms. When estrogen goes up, progesterone is supposed to go down.

We know what normal FUNCTION is. What we don't know is this: Why is a woman having symptoms—not functioning normally—when there is no pathology? Trying to figure this out was a puzzle wrapped in a mystery and surrounded by a conundrum.

What was throwing everything off? Was PMS related to nutrition, or a lack of it? After all, in my practice I've often

CHAPTER 1—Cracking the Code: *The Difference Proper Nutrition Makes*

said that I don't treat disease. Many studies have convincingly proven that PMS is not a disease.

That's what I was looking for back in 1980.

If I could just find one commonality among PMS sufferers.

The moment was at hand, though it had been a long time coming on a long learning curve.

> To understand how nutrition can help ease the symptoms of PMS, we first need to understand a bit of physiology. Once you know how everything is connected, you can make nutritional choices to bring your menstrual cycle back into balance. It's important to pause here and really get into how the body works. If menstruation is necessary for reproduction, which is a normal function of your body, why are you having symptoms?
>
> **Menstruation is not a disease.**

The Nutrition Key

I first became interested in nutrition during my chiropractic training at Logan College in St. Louis, where we received the same basic education over a five-year period as any medical doctor received at that time—anatomy, physiology, biochemistry, pathology, microbiology, and so on. The medical doctor then goes after drug therapy and function, and the chiropractor goes after structure.

Or that's the way chiropractic has come to be perceived, as dealing exclusively with structure.

In fact, this is only half the equation. Back in the 1960s, we were taught chiropractic as it was originally conceived—as a three-dimensional healing art combining both the visceral and structural aspects of the human body.

> The development of this integrated system begins during the third week (16th day) of human embryonic development, when the nervous system, the internal organs and the musculoskeletal system grow out of three distinct "primary embryonic layers."

The outer layer, or ectoderm, evolves to become the skin, the hair, the nails, the upper respiratory tract, and the brain and spinal cord. The middle layer, or mesoderm, becomes the musculoskeletal system, the body's connective tissues, the circulatory system and the lymphatic system. The innermost layer, or endoderm, forms the body's working organs.

While all this is taking place, the spinal cord is sending out nerve fibers, connecting these three layers to receptors in the skin, the muscles, and all the organs of the body. It is through this hard-wired "neuro-switchboard" that the brain will receive and send messages, regulating all body functions in times of normalcy and in times of stress.

When an organ is struggling and sends a distress signal to the brain, the returning message goes to all three layers or tissues, the skin, the muscles, and the involved organ. They all respond even though only one is sending the distress signal. Hence, a struggling gall bladder can trigger involuntary muscle contractions around the shoulder.

And so, as a chiropractor, I learned that pain in a patient's shoulder may have nothing to do with a structural injury to that shoulder. The pain may actually result from a visceral cause—the outward expression of a stressed gallbladder or other organ having trouble doing its job. All the manipulation or physical therapy in the world will not make this pain go away permanently. It will be back with the next meal.

Early Researchers, Remarkable Discoveries

This is precisely the vision that D.D. Palmer had when he founded the field of chiropractic in 1895, two years after he performed the first chiropractic adjustment on a partially deaf janitor, Harvey Lillard. After the adjustment, Harvey said that he could actually hear the sound of horses in the street. I had just such an experience after a chiropractic adjustment during my own hearing-impaired youth.

Two prominent researchers whose early work gave rise to this three-dimensional thinking were Henry Head and James MacKenzie.

Sir Henry Head was one of the principal developers of clinical neuroscience, which included the mapping out of human dermatomes—areas of the skin served by sensory neurons rooted in the spinal cord. Studying patients suffering from shingles, Head was able to trace their surface pain directly to its corresponding roots in their spinal nerves, with the specific area of the skin experiencing the pain corresponding to a specific section of the spinal cord.

This work was published in 1900.

Furthermore, Head found that diseases involving the internal organs can produce these same surface symptoms and other "tender areas" when impulses from the brain are sent out along the shared "party line." Anytime an organ is under stress and not functioning properly, measurable changes will occur on the skin, according to Head. That's what his mapping of human dermatomes revealed.

Then there was Sir James MacKenzie, a Scottish cardiologist known for his pioneering work in cardiac arrhythmias. MacKenzie noted in 1917 that there are two kinds of muscle contractions occurring in the human body—voluntary and involuntary. Voluntary muscle contractions are associated with specific body functions (e.g., the scratching of one's nose); involuntary muscle contractions (e.g., the twitching of an eye), he called "visceral-motor reflexes."

Unlike voluntary contractions, MacKenzie found, involuntary contractions do not necessarily result in a shortening of the muscle. Nor do they necessarily involve the entire length of the muscle. Further, an involuntary muscle contraction is not subject to fatigue, so it can last for an indefinite time.

Therfore the struggling gallbladder can produce chronic shoulder pain.

This how a chiropractor can distinguish between a structural or visceral cause of involuntary muscle contractions.

What I found in the first few months of my practice was that most of the musculoskeletal complaints coming my way were, in fact, visceral in origin. An organ—the stomach, gallbladder, pancreas, prostate, uterus, breast, whatever—was not doing what it was supposed to do, because the organ was under stress.

And that stress was causing an involuntary muscle contraction, which caused loss of range of motion in the joint.

This is where chiropractic really captured my imagination. Because it had to do with Universal Intelligence.

What Is Universal Intelligence?

Universal Intelligence has been described as "the intrinsic tendency for things to self-organize and co-evolve into ever more complex, intricately interwoven and mutually compatible forms."

> **On a more personal note, one might say that each of us is a universe unto ourselves, with every cellular aspect of our life functions orchestrated by the same Universal Intelligence that has done so in all living creatures since the beginning of time.**

We think again of the switchboard and all its components. The image illustrates the Universal Intelligence that enables all our body cells and organ systems to function as intended, in harmony, to do their individual part—their job—in maintaining homeostasis.

It's All About Maintaining Homeostasis

The word homeostasis was first coined by the American physiologist Walter B. Cannon in 1930 from the Greek words "same" and "steady" to describe how the human body maintains an internal environment conducive to the healthy functioning of all its cells. Certain fundamental activities represent the minimal requirements for maintaining cell integrity and life. These activities include the following:

- Take food from the surrounding environment and excrete waste back into that environment.
- Produce energy by breaking down nutrients and making new molecules from them.
- Reproduce.
- Consistently demonstrate the will to live.

It is the extracellular fluid, in which all body cells live and breathe, so to speak, which acts as a nutritional delivery and waste removal system.

Think of it this way: 60 percent of the human body weight is water. The fluid inside the cells (intracellular fluid) accounts for two-thirds of the total body water. The fluid outside the cells (extracellular fluid) accounts for the other third. This extracellular fluid must remain relatively constant in terms of acid-alkaline balance (pH), temperature, volume (the amount of water) and levels of dissolved substances needed to nourish the cells, such as sugar, protein, cholesterol and iron. And calcium, as we will soon see.

Homeostasis must be maintained if cells and organ systems are to function in a healthy manner.

It is the job of the body's 10 organ systems—the circulatory, digestive, endocrine, immune, integumentary (skin), musculoskeletal, nervous, reproductive, respiratory and urinary—to provide and maintain this internal environment and act as a life-support system for all the body's individual cells.

At the Controls

The body has two major control systems for maintaining homeostasis.

The autonomic, or involuntary nervous system, controls things like heart rate, digestion, respiratory rate, salivation, perspiration, sexual arousal, and so on.

Then there's the endocrine system—the glands that secret hormones. These include the pituitary gland; the pancreas, which also secretes digestive enzymes into the digestive tract; the ovaries; the thyroid gland; the testes; and the adrenal glands.

Both these systems—autonomic and endocrine—receive signals and direction from the brain, more specifically from the hypothalamus, which is seated just above the brain stem.

When it comes to maintaining homeostasis, the hypothalamus pretty much runs the show.

But when it comes to troops on the ground, protein is king.

About Protein

There are two kinds of protein in the body. There's protein that cells use for growth and repair, which can also be converted into energy. And there are the blood-borne plasma proteins, which maintain homeostasis. Plasma proteins transport nutrients; they detoxify waste; they maintain pH by buffering excess acidity or alkalinity; and they maintain the fluid balance in the extracellular fluid.

It's protein that maintains calcium in the blood. At any given time, roughly 50 percent of the calcium in the blood will be free-floating, while 50 percent will be bound to protein. When excess calcium shows up in the urine, this can be a sign of protein deficiency, because the brain will dump calcium to maintain the 50/50 ratio between free-floating calcium and calcium bound to protein.

This protein-calcium relationship is key to understanding PMS, as we will soon see.

Maintaining homeostasis in extracellular fluids is the number one priority for the Universal Intelligence that is born into each and every one of us. Any deviation produces organ stress, and eventually disease. When it comes to maintaining homeostasis, stress is the enemy.

Stress: The Universal Enemy

I learned this in the late 1960s, during my chiropractic training, with the release of Hans Selye's landmark book, *The Stress of Life*. That book, followed by 1,700 research papers over four decades, earned Selye eight Nobel Prize nominations and the acclaim of all those in the healing arts.

Selye proved that the human body responds to any kind of stress, be it mechanical, chemical or emotional, in a very specific and predictable way.

Selye called this response the "general adaptation syndrome." It starts with the body in a state of health, or normalcy. If a "stimulus stress" is applied that requires a change to maintain normalcy, a signal is sent to the brain, which in turn sends out signals producing a resistance reaction. If the stimulus disappears and was not strong enough to disrupt normal function, then we probably don't even notice the reaction that has taken place.

Many such reactions occur every day as we adjust our rates of respiration and heartbeat, as well as countless hormonal and autonomic nerve responses, to meet changes and challenges in our environment—both external and internal.

If the stimulus stress continues, those parts of the body affected must elicit aid from other tissues, or use more energy-producing nutrients to maintain their heightened state of function. This situation will continue without issue, as long as the flow of nutrition is maintained and the waste products produced by the affected organ/tissue are transported away and not allowed to accumulate.

However, once tissues under stress become fatigued because of a lack of continuing support from related tissues or organs, nutrition or waste removal, or because the stimulus is simply too strong, we enter a state of exhaustion.

It is at this point that we begin to experience symptoms. Fortunately, the affected tissues are not exhausted to the point of damage. Objective findings—from physical examination (except for palpation of involuntary muscle contractions and alterations on a 24-hour urine sample), blood tests, and X-rays—are still negative. We have not yet reached the point of disease.

And yet, health has not been maintained.

> **The question now becomes, which way do we move next—up to health or down to disease, degeneration and eventually death?**

Selye's findings demonstrate that since the human body has its own specific ways of maintaining normal function, and therefore health, any healing attempts should be directed at relieving the stress and providing the nutrients for the body to use in its own defense—and its own healing process.

Such efforts, in conjunction with removing excessive waste that always results when cells are stressed and stimulated, would fall within the province of nutrition.

And so, for Selye, the best way to treat a body under stress is to provide the right nutrition to restore homeostasis and normal function to the stressed organs or organ systems, before the body reaches a state of disease.

The Wheel Comes Full Circle

This is where I placed my efforts when I first put up my chiropractic shingle—looking for ways to diagnose and relieve visceral issues via nutrition.

I had my tools.

First was the taking of the patient's history. What kind of emotional stress were they going through that might produce a weakness in the body? What kind of injuries or surgeries had they been through? What kinds of medications were they taking that might produce their symptom, or be camouflaging the underlying problem?

CHAPTER 1—Cracking the Code: *The Difference Proper Nutrition Makes*

Then came the physical exam—listening to the heart and lungs; looking at things like head tilt, or whether the shoulders and hips are level; looking at knee flexion and ankle pronation. Looking for involuntary muscle contractions that might signal a structural or visceral issue.

The visceral issues were the most vexing—trying to figure out the source of the muscle contraction. What organ or organs were struggling in doing their part to maintain homeostasis?

What was the nutritional deficiency?

The 24-hour urinalysis was a key tool for tracking down deficiencies. If there wasn't any calcium showing up in a patient's urine over a 24-hour period, as it should be, I would know that the body is calcium deficient. If it's eliminating more calcium that it should be, that may mean it doesn't have enough protein to hold onto the calcium, and the patient is protein deficient.

Then there were the blood tests, which are used to measure inflammation. Add an anticoagulant to a blood sample and set it aside for 24 hours. During that time, the red blood cells separate from the serum and fall to the bottom. The faster they fall, the more inflamed the patient is.

So urine and blood tests were good for detecting various deficiencies.

The question then became, how do you correct such deficiencies once you are able to identify them?

Restoring Health

For the next 12 years, I would endeavor to use all my tools to identify the nutritional deficiencies causing my patients' visceral symptoms, and then to nourish their bodies with the vitamin and mineral supplements at my disposal, and finally to restore function and health.

That was my mission.

The town I practiced in had less than 1,000 residents. Forsyth was a Civil War-era town, a winding drive east through the monumental Ozarks from the "micropolitan" music mecca that is Branson, Missouri. There were no unions, no industry to speak of. Many of the people living in Forsyth were retired and living on fixed incomes. There were no salad bars, no health food stores. Anybody taking vitamins or supplements was considered a "health nut." This was because the pharmaceutical companies and the medical doctors were claiming that there was no benefit to vitamin and mineral supplementation.

Then in 1965 Adelle Davis's book, *Let's Get Well*, was published, and the industry started taking off. Pharmaceutical companies were buying up supplement companies and touting their products for everything under the sun, sometimes at the expense of public health.

A chiropractor in a rural area like Forsyth doesn't specialize in injury or structural problems only. Mine was a general practice. People struggling with a multitude of general-practice symptoms and unable to get relief would come to me. People with sinus trouble, bladder issues, urinary problems, digestive problems. Everything came through my door. My biggest responsibility was determining whether there was pathology involved and if so to refer that person for appropriate medical treatment.

But if I could discover through examination and blood and urine testing that a patient had a nutritional deficiency underlying their symptoms, I would go after that deficiency.

My first foray was into intervertebral discs.

The problem with these discs, which provide shock absorption and range of motion for the spine, is that they can become thin or degenerate. Each disc has a liquid center, which is made up of water and protein. It's the protein that holds the water in a jelly-like suspension and maintains the integrity of the disc. Without the protein, the water will dissipate and the disc will thin. The patient will experience stress, pain, and loss of flexibility in the spine.

I reasoned that patients with thinned-out discs might be having a problem with protein metabolism, and hence a protein deficiency.

If I could just get more protein metabolized and absorbed into their spine.

Betaine HCl was widely used by the pharmaceutical industry at the time and incorrectly described as improving protein digestion. That, I figured (incorrectly), would improve protein assimilation.

There were the protein supplements. Spirulina was a good one.

I also had ox bile salts to (theoretically) help improve the flow of bile, to aid the breaking down of fats, and the absorption of vitamins A, D, E and K, all for good measure.

And I had pancreatic (animal) enzymes that would facilitate more complete digestion of the protein.

I was all set to be the next 90-day wonder.

Unfortunately, I could never get any improvement in the blood and urine tests—there was no detectable improvement in protein assimilation. The protein wasn't being properly digested.

I wasn't getting any significant improvement in joint range of motion in the spines of my patients either.

That was just one approach. Over the next 12 years, I used everything under the kitchen sink—all manner of supplements, including vitamins and minerals—as well as manipulating people's diets. But nothing worked. There was no evidence of any consistent, reliable benefit with regard to any symptom or cluster of symptoms. Just like PMS.

I could adjust and get relief for my patients, but the relief wouldn't last if the source was visceral.

I eventually came to realize that vitamin and mineral supplements don't work because they are not food. They're chemicals. They are refined down to a single ingredient for pharmaceutical nutrition. That's what drugs are based on.

By definition, food is something that contains protein, carbohydrate, lipids, vitamins and minerals, and other substances. For example, 500 milligrams of vitamin C is a drug; it's not food. But it's not a very strong drug, or it would require a prescription.

The body just doesn't know what to do with them. This has played out in recent studies demonstrating the lack of benefit in some vitamin and mineral supplements for specific symptoms.

I became interested in herbs as whole food sources. Still nothing in terms of any therapeutic benefit I could count on.

Something in my equation was clearly missing.

Enter Dr. Howell

Then Tony Collier showed up at my door with his line of plant enzyme supplements. Collier had recently relocated the National Enzyme Company, founded by Dr. Edward Howell in 1932 as a small mail-order operation, to Forsyth. He had bought the entire complex next door and was setting up manufacturing, hoping for national and ultimately global sales.

Howell's interest in plant enzyme supplements grew out of his early discovery that the natural enzymes contained in the foods we eat, which Nature intended to assist us in our digestion of these foods, are destroyed in the cooking process, and during pasteurization.

Basically, heat kills these "food enzymes"—protease, which digests protein; lipase, which digests fats; amylase, which digests carbohydrates; and cellulase, which digests plant fibers.

The absence of these food enzymes, Howell theorized, places a larger than normal burden on the human pancreas to produce enough enzymes (all but cellulase, which the human body does not produce) to digest everything in our enzyme-deficient cooked and processed food diet.

The inability of the human pancreas to meet this demand, Howell wrote in *Enzyme Nutrition: The Food Enzyme Concept*, results in the accumulation and putrefaction of partially digested foods in the large intestine, and an inflammatory cascade responsible for many of the chronic diseases afflicting humankind today—from arthritis and diabetes to heart disease and cancer.

In contrast, these widespread chronic diseases are not commonly found among carnivores and herbivores that live in the wild and eat enzyme-rich raw foods, as Nature originally intended.

That was Howell's theory.

And that's what led him to plant enzyme supplements as a means of replacing the missing food enzymes in the human diet, and achieving more complete digestion. Actually, the more appropriate term is predigestion, because food enzymes do their digestive work in the upper part of the stomach, or the "food enzyme stomach," as Howell called it. That's before the food is acted upon by protein-digesting pepsin in the lower stomach, and pancreatic enzymes in the small intestine.

Many have dismissed food enzymes as not being strong enough to do any real digestive work, or questioned their ability to survive the hydrochloric acid in the stomach. Both of these assertions have been proven not true. Animal and human studies have shown that food enzymes are strong enough to perform these predigestive duties. Furthermore, stomach acid is not created in the stomach until at least half an hour after a meal begins, giving food enzymes plenty of time to do their work.

My issue, when Collier came to my door, was not whether food enzymes would assist in digestion. I knew they would. I was more concerned whether the work they do would help relieve my patient's symptoms, with any consistency.

> **"Work" is the key word here. The ability to perform work is the definition of energy. Vitamins and minerals do not perform work. It's enzymes that provide the energy to put these vitamins and minerals to work. They are the driving force behind every body function. Enzymes are, in Howell's words, Nature's workers.**

Could food enzymes help me deliver specific types of nutrition to struggling organ systems? Perhaps.

I decided to start off with a product containing a blend of plant-derived protease, lipase, amylase and cellulase. I'd tried this blend before, with insufficient improvement in digestion and no effect on urinalysis and blood tests. So I had Collier boost the potency—the "activity level"—of the blend.

He made me 100 bottles, which I gave to 100 patients, instructing them to take two capsules with each meal for 30 days. These patients had a variety of problems, primarily structural, such as joint pain, back pain, elbow pain, as well as headaches, digestive problems, and so on.

After 30 days, patients said they felt much better. They could digest their food better, and they slept better. They all wanted more. But I was unable to determine from examinations, and from blood and urine tests, how to use the plant enzymes.

There was no common denominator, no commonality.

That's when I decided to take a different course and work with just one plant enzyme at a time. I asked Collier to make me one pure dose of protease so I could study them one at a time.

And make it stronger.

This time I had my patients take the capsules between meals. With no food in the stomach, the protease enzymes could make it right into the small intestine where they could be absorbed into the body and sent wherever they were needed.

I got lucky. I was finding areas where there seemed to be diminished bone pain—weight-bearing areas that are under physical stress. The shins, in particular, which take a lot of punishment when someone runs on concrete or asphalt. So patients with shin splints were having less pain.

I had Collier double the dose again. This time, urinalysis revealed that my patients were becoming slightly calcium deficient. Meanwhile, more protease meant more complete digestion of protein, and bone is made up of protein.

So what I was seeing in these patients told me that protease enzymes were good for relieving shin pain.

Finally, something I could depend on consistently.

It was at that point that an article I'd read in the Scientific American led me to believe there might be something in this protease approach for the chronic ear infections that had wrought havoc on my own life for the past 40 years.

I was 10 months old when an attack of whooping cough took away half my hearing.

Whooping cough was a terror back in 1938. Caused by the highly contagious Bordetella pertussis bacteria, whooping cough typically starts with mild symptoms that gradually develop into severe coughing fits of five to 10 forceful coughs, marked by the high-pitched "whoop" sound as the infant or child inhales air after coughing. The coughing stage usually lasts about six weeks before subsiding. In some cases, the child does not survive.

We were living in Dunkirk, New York, on the banks of Lake Erie. My mother and my father's mother, both nurses, cared for me, giving me the gold shots the doctor had ordered before running from the house. Penicillin wouldn't be introduced until after World War II, though the best that antibiotics would ever offer in the case of active whooping cough would be to shorten the infectious stage of the disease.

I was quarantined. My father, the town baker, was forbidden to enter my room.

There were times when my mother did not expect me to live. I did survive, but those big whoops had knocked out my hearing in both ears, leaving me with between 40 and 50 percent of normal hearing range, and persistently draining middle ear infections. I endured excruciating earaches in both ears that would never let up, and both my ears were continuously draining pus.

Every year, I missed a half year of school as I lay in bed for weeks, my ears throbbing with pain. At 13, I had my tonsils out, and the worst of those earaches disappeared. But the infections remained as a continuous, purulent draining out of both ears, which is why I was not able to wear a hearing aid. Nothing could go inside my ears because of those infections.

The only thing in school that saved me was that I could read. I owe my life to my sixth-grade teacher, Mrs. Clark, who realized how well I could read and introduced me to the library, to the dictionary and the card catalog. I was reading Carl Sandburg's *Life of Lincoln* that summer.

That book set me up for the rest of my life.

My big break came in 1955, when I learned about the bone conduction hearing aid, which fit on a pair of glasses and pressed up against the bone behind the ear, with sounds being transmitted clearly through these bones. Suddenly, my hearing was testing at 110 percent.

And so my hearing life began, though the chronic draining ear infections continued. The only thing that ever touched them was the antibacterial drug Gantrisin, which was approved in 1950. The doctor had to give me a double shot in the buttocks, along with the oral dose, for the ear infection to stop. But as soon as I got any water in my ears, the infection returned.

The chiropractor was the only other person who helped me. He'd lay me face down and get his thumb under the bottom part of my sacrum, the tail bone, and he'd elevate me as he went up my spine, manipulating every bone, looking for muscle contractions.

It worked every time. It slowed down the drainage and some of the inflammation, and my hearing improved.

And yet, those draining infections continued, right up to the day Tony Collier came to my door in Forsyth with his pre-digestive plant enzymes.

It was the aforementioned article in the *Scientific American* that got me thinking that Collier's protease enzymes might work on my chronic ear infections. I'd read the article back in 1967. It described how disease-fighting white blood cells kill bacteria and viruses by injecting them with protease enzymes. Inside each white blood cell is a lysosome package containing protease enzymes. Illustrations showed how a white blood cell gets

CHAPTER 1—Cracking the Code: *The Difference Proper Nutrition Makes*

belly to belly with a bacteria, and how it uses calcium as a trigger to literally shoot the protease into the bacteria, which are then destroyed.

Once again, it was just a matter of getting the protease enzymes across the intestinal wall and into the bloodstream so they could be delivered where they were needed.

And once again, I asked Collier to double the dose.

He did so, and I began taking the capsules between meals.

Two or three days passed. Nothing happened.

"Double it again," I said.

"Okay, but be careful," he said. He hadn't made anything that strong before.

And I took them. This time I got a rip-roaring pain in my ears. My ears felt literally on fire with inflammation.

I knew I was on the right track. My fully armed immune cells were on the attack. But it wasn't enough. I needed more enzymes!

Collier was reluctant, but once again, he upped the dose.

And I took some calcium with it.

It stopped it cold. Within 36 hours, the infection that I had lived with for 43 years was gone. And it never came back.

Though I was able to wear an inside-the-ear hearing aid for the first time in my life, I was still not much better off in my understanding of how to use plant enzymes and other dietary supplements to relieve my patients' visceral symptoms. That understanding would come to me over the next five years.

That was the new approach I was offering when the five women suffering from PMS symptoms came to my office in October 1980.

Nutritional Deficiencies and PMS

During my first 12 years in practice, I saw a lot of young women under a lot of emotional stress—struggling to pay the bills, raising their children and trying to maintain happy households.

Every month they would be stuck with this menstrual cycle and all these symptoms—everything from irritability to abdominal cramps. Some women couldn't get out of bed for several days. Headaches were common, moodiness, and the amount of flow, which could range from very light one month to a deluge of bleeding the next. Fatigue, exhaustion, back pain—there was no end to it. And everyone's experience was different.

There was just no rhyme or reason to PMS. There still isn't. You sit there and listen to all of this and try to figure out what's causing it. You feel sorry for the patient's discomfort. You do the best you can to help, but there's no help to offer—only temporary symptomatic relief.

I could relieve back pain with a chiropractic adjustment. It's all coming from the nerves in the lower back that go into the uterus and the ovaries. And from pelvic misalignment.

I could treat headaches associated with PMS. They're basically muscle tension headaches. You just adjust between the shoulder blades and the neck.

But the back pain and headaches, and a lot more, will all return with the next monthly cycle.

Now I had plant enzymes. What I was interested in was not treating symptoms, but finding some commonality, if it existed, and going with that.

This opportunity presented itself when the five women who came to my office during those two weeks in October 1980 agreed to undergo the necessary tests, at my expense of course, to determine how to use this new approach I had in mind.

I started out with the examination, doing a patient history, looking for stress in their lives, how many children they had, and looking for involuntary muscle contractions.

Then came the blood tests and 24-hour urine testing.

What I was looking for showed up in the urine—an absence of calcium. All five women were not putting enough calcium into the urine. In other words, the body didn't have enough calcium to throw away. It was hoarding it.

All five women were calcium deficient!

And their urine was very alkaline, which told me they weren't digesting enough protein, which creates acidity.

So it struck me that if I could increase acidity through digesting protein—and add a little calcium to their diet—that should theoretically work in terms of relieving some of these symptoms.

And sure enough, with protease enzymes to digest protein in the stomach, and a small amount of supplemental calcium, all of these women's urine patterns changed over the next couple of weeks, as did their symptom patterns.

All five patients were now excreting normal amounts of calcium in their urine on a day-to-day basis, indicating that they were no longer calcium deficient. And they were no longer alkaline. Their pH was more balanced between acidity and alkalinity. This was all measured in their urinalyses.

Further, muscle contraction patterns associated with acid deficiency went away as well.

Specific muscle contractions related to calcium deficiency also went away, especially in the lower back.

Also dramatically improved was muscle cramping in the pelvis associated with PMS, which is related to calcium deficiency, as well as muscle contraction patterns due to structural misalignment caused by these cramps.

Back pain and headache were both improved, as was irritability. As you become more calcium deficient you become more irritable.

Joint pain also improved.

And because we were combining calcium with protease enzymes, which improved protein absorption, some of the edema, or bloating, associated with PMS was going away. This is because when you are protein deficient, water leaves the blood and accumulates in body tissues.

In all five women, these symptoms improved.

I was on Cloud 9!

Two weeks after their periods, the women's urine tests were still looking good, and I was thinking they wouldn't have any PMS symptoms when their next period arrived. But that wasn't the case. Their symptoms were back.

I was deeply disappointed, and so were they.

But when they got their next period, the symptoms did not reappear. They were back to normal. And as long as they stayed on the program, their PMS symptoms did not reappear.

To me, it was like a miracle. I remember thinking, it can't be that simple. But it was.

It literally put tears in my eyes.

I treated thousands of women similarly in the years that followed. I was never able to get it totally correct by the next period, or explain why the relapse into symptoms; but, by the second period, in most cases, the women were back to normal.

Protease enzymes were the key. Women tend to be protein deficient. And protein and calcium are homeostatically linked.

This was my foray into women's nutrition. And I must say it changed my way of thinking. I went from wishing I could simply write a prescription for an antidepressant to wishing I could have a practice devoted entirely to women's health. I had cracked the code.

Why? Because in my experience women are far more motivated, and far more willing, to change their habits than men are. As a result, the chances for success are much greater.

CHAPTER 2

In the Beginning

From Childhood to Puberty

So when did Eve become Eve?

According to ancient Judeo-Christian-Muslim literature, Eve was never a child, never a maiden—*(never went through puberty)*. On the day she was created, she emerged from Adam a fully developed woman with all her "procreative abilities" intact.

Some argue that Adam had no gender until Eve's emergence, at which point sexual differentiation began, with Eve becoming "the mother of all living."

After eating the forbidden fruit, the two were cast out of Eden to a land where Adam and his male descendants would toil among the thorns while Eve and all her female descendants would suffer the pains of conception, which has been broadly interpreted to include all aspects of procreation, beginning at menarche—a woman's first menstrual cycle—continuing through pregnancy and culminating in the pain of childbirth. But, as we now know, it all begins with menarche.

Menarche: A Rite of Passage

This rite of passage, which comes without warning and varies in age of onset from individual to individual, marks the moment at which the female child becomes a fertile woman.

In many cultures, menarche is celebrated as a time of divine empowerment, with rituals commemorating the young woman's entry into maidenhood.

Moroccans throw the young woman a lavish party and shower her with money and gifts.

Young Dyak women in Southeast Asia spend a contemplative year secluded in a white cabin, wearing white clothes and eating white foods believed to promote good health. During this time, they are visited by elder women who counsel and instruct them in the art of womanhood. All this is done not out of fear but in reverence.

"One of the most beautiful examples of menarche initiation," Elizabeth Davis writes in her essay on "The Menarche Rite," "is the Apache rite of 'Changing Woman.' "

In this ceremony, Davis writes, the pubescent girl becomes "the primordial Apache mother," the "White Painted Woman," reenacting the story of how the Changing Woman became "impregnated by the sun" and "gave birth to the Apache people."

The ritual lasts four days.

"On the first day," Davis writes, "she is sprinkled with yellow cattail pollen to symbolize fertility, and is taught by wise-women of the 'fire-within,' her sacred sexuality."

On the final night, the woman dances from sunset to sunrise "for the well-being of her people."

At dawn, a song is sung to her:

"Now you are entering the world ...You will become an adult with responsibilities ... Walk with honor and dignity ... Be strong! ... For you are the mother of our people ... For you will become the mother of a nation."

China's Taoists and the Ancient Egyptians consumed menstrual blood mixed with red wine to increase their spiritual power.

In ancient Greece, spring festivals included the spreading of corn mixed with menstrual blood to increase the soil's fertility.

Then there's the other side of the coin.

In some societies, ancient myths attribute menarche and the subsequent emotional and physiologic changes that accompany it to a curse resulting from Eve's collaboration with the serpent.

In Ethiopia, Beta Jewish women are regarded as impure when they are menstruating and are isolated from the male population in menstruation huts built near bodies of water so that they may cleanse themselves.

Some religions prohibit menstruating women from entering temples because they are seen as being religiously unclean.

Given its social and physical implications, menarche and the ensuing menstrual cycle is probably best characterized as a mixed blessing, but a blessing nonetheless. Nutrition, as we will see, is a leading factor in which way and how far the pendulum will swing, with regard to symptoms both physical and emotional.

Menstruation

Menstruation is what separates men from women. It's what makes women more emotional and more sensitive to stress—the hormonal shifts that occur during menstruation.

And it all begins at menarche, with the emergence of this new emotional self.

Young women have come to my office confounded.

"It seemed like this was the first time I found myself crying without having a clue why," one patient told me. "It was the start of the emotional roller coaster and the feeling that something was wrong with me mentally because I couldn't control it or find a reason for it."

Young women today are full of optimism, and worry.

How will my body develop?

Will I ever have breasts? My friends have breasts already, and I have nothing at age 16!

Will I have a good figure?

There has always been the belief that a good figure will change a woman's station and identity in life. Females today are under even more pressure and expectations. The social pressure to fit the image of the "ideal woman" has a large impact on the way young girls and women view their bodies—trying to live up to the images they see in magazines and television. Eating disorders have become extremely prevalent.

Stress starts at a much earlier age today, as parents put their children on a fast track starting in preschool.

Then menarche hits.

All of a sudden progesterone shoots sky high and estrogen begins to level out and drop. That's ovulation. Once that hits, the mother is gradually going to begin to notice that her daughter, who has been difficult to deal with anyway, is becoming irritable and anxious and crying for no reason.

From a woman's first ovulation, her life will never be entirely her own again. For many, the words "Tell me I'm not crazy" will reverberate with each recurring visit to her doctor and each new prescription for antidepressants.

Unlike her male counterpart, the woman's reproductive system is the most significant factor in determining how she will be treated, not only in the area of health care but in other areas as well. Today, many women view their menstrual cycle with displeasure—that monthly bleeding is such a nuisance.

For others, there is no issue at all.

Phases of the Moon

One of the most fascinating subjects I came across while preparing for a seminar on women's health and nutrition was the concept that there is an intimate emotional connection between a woman's cycle and the phases of the moon. When I mentioned this to women attending the seminar, many agreed, while others thought the idea ridiculous. One thing they all agreed upon, however, and which I myself was familiar, was the reported phenomenon concerning women grouped together for extended lengths of time beginning to synchronize their menstrual cycles.

While I found the whole concept quite bewildering, I decided to look at the possibility of the variations in hormonal balance during a menstrual cycle and compare them to the emotional cycle described by Christiane Northrup, M.D., in her book, *Women's Bodies, Women's Wisdom*.

Again, keeping in mind that estrogen is a central nervous system stimulant, while progesterone has a depressing effect on the central nervous system.

Northrup describes the menstrual cycle as "the most basic earthly cycle we have," comparing it to the "macrocosmic cycles of Nature, the waxing and waning [of the moon], the ebb and flow of the tides and the changes of the seasons." All these, she contends, "are reflected on a smaller scale in the menstrual cycle of the individual female body," while the "monthly ripening of an egg and subsequent pregnancy or release of menstrual blood mirror the process of creation as it occurs not only in Nature ... but in human endeavor."

Thus menarche becomes a sacred rite of passage for every woman in harmony with all of Nature going back to Eve. Recent studies, Northrup notes, show that "peak rates of conception and probably ovulation appear to occur at the full moon or the day before."

The same can be said of a woman's emotions and creativity, as the phases of her cycle are related to the corresponding phases of the lunar cycle.

During the "New Moon," which corresponds to the "New Menstrual Cycle," estradiol (estrogen produced by the ovaries) is rising.

NORTHRUP: "We start a new cycle and have more energy and are more extroverted."

During the "Waxing Moon," when estradiol continues to rise, then sharply declines.

NORTHRUP: "We brim with creativity and are action oriented, anxious to fuel our ideas."

During the "Next Full Moon," progesterone spikes.

NORTHRUP: Our creativity peaks with ovulation. This is the fertile time, or time for creating new life within our body. Many women find that their sexual energy is heightened at this time, as it is Nature's time to reproduce."

During the "Waning Moon," both estrogen and progesterone have leveled off and begin a slow decline towards menstruation.

NORTHRUP: "As the full moon wanes and our ovulation is completed, women move into an inner reflective stage." This phase between ovulation and menstruation is a time "when women are most in tune with their inner knowing and with what isn't working in their lives." It is a time when women are much more emotional. It is during this reflective phase that women tend to dwell on the negative aspects of their lives and are "more apt to cry."

It is this phase of the cycle that has become known as "premenstrual syndrome," or PMS.

"Finally," Northrup writes, "during the final stages of the waning moon our bleeding begins. It is a time for deep reflection, a time to nurture ourselves, to slow down and be quiet as our bodies release."

And so the moon cycles metaphorically within the menstruating female mind and body.

And yet, the cycle remains shrouded in mystery as the dark side of the moon makes it unpredictable—from when it will begin to how much it will impact a woman's physical and emotional being.

This is where nutrition comes in—and stress.

So What's Normal?

The normal menstrual period is 28 days, give or take 3 days, for 65 percent of women, with a range of 18 to 40 days. Once a menstrual pattern has been established, the variation does not normally exceed five days. The average duration of flow is five days, give or take two days, with a blood loss averaging 130 milliliters, with flow generally heaviest on the second day.
Then there's not normal.

Amenorrhea, or the absence of a menstrual cycle, falls into three broad categories.

Women with primary amenorrhea do not begin to menstruate when expected. Because there is a wide variation in normal onset of menstruation during puberty, applying this diagnosis is problematic. In general, however, primary amenorrhea implies that menstruation has not yet started by the age of 16.

Treatment could begin at the age of 15, if deemed necessary. However, a competent diagnosis is required, as there are a number of diverse causes to consider, including imperforate hymen, ovarian dysfunction, and hormonal imbalance—or fat deficiency, as we will see.

Find the cause and the treatment becomes obvious.

There are no magic bullets for secondary amenorrhea. In this case, the diagnosis is made with cessation of menstruation after at least one normal period. Secondary amenorrhea is fairly common. Causes include: stress, loss or gain of weight, anemia, excessive exercise, discontinuation of oral contraceptives, ovarian cysts and some tumors.

Erratic or irregular menstruation, whereby a woman may have three or four periods a year, or three very close periods followed by none for several months, has numerous causes, similar to those resulting in secondary amenorrhea.

Dysmenorrhea, or painful menstruation, is the most common of all gynecologic complaints and the leading cause of absenteeism of women from school, work, and other activities. In addition to identifiable pathological causes, a number of constitutional factors may lower an individual's pain threshold and thus appear to worsen dysmenorrhea. These factors include anemia, increase in obesity, chronic illness, overwork, stress, diabetes, and poor nutrition.

Primary Dysmenorrhea is unrelated to any pelvic lesions, and most often starts with the first ovulation cycle. Fifty percent of patients experience nausea, 25 percent experience vomiting, 35 percent have increased stool frequency. The pain is low and cramping, recurring in waves that probably correlate with uterine contractions. The pain usually begins a few hours before bleeding commences, comes to peak intensity within a few hours, and dissipates within two days. It generally occurs over the midline of the abdomen, and is relieved by the onset of menstrual flow.

Secondary Dysmenorrhea is related to the presence of pelvic lesions associated with organic pelvic disease, such as endometriosis, pelvic inflammatory disease, and post-surgical adhesions. The contraceptive intrauterine device (IUD) may cause pain problems.

Secondary dysmenorrhea begins up to a few days before menstruation and lasts several days after the onset of flow.

Often it is lateralized to one side of the body, and it does not characteristically peak and diminish as clearly or quickly as primary dysmenorrhea. In general, the onset of secondary dysmenorrhea occurs later in life.

A big player in all of the above menstrual issues is stress, and a lack of energy for body organs under stress—particularly those of the reproductive/endocrine systems—to maintain normal function and do their part in maintaining homeostasis.

Stress = Energy Deficiencies

Like Selye demonstrated, sources of stress can be emotional, chemical, or structural. It doesn't matter what the source is, stress is stress, and it takes energy for the body to deal with it. So where does the body get its energy?

The human body has three sources of energy: carbohydrates, protein and fat (lipids), and it uses them in that order.

The body prefers carbohydrates as its primary source of glucose to supply energy. When the body runs out of carbohydrates, it turns to protein as its second source of glucose, and finally to stored fat.

Carbohydrate is the first choice because it's easily converted into energy by all cells.

However, carbohydrates are not stored widely in the body—only in the liver and the muscles, as an emergency source of energy. While muscles store glucose, in the form of glycogen, this can only be used by the muscles in the event of a "fight or flight" situation, where there is an acute demand for energy to meet an emergency.

When the body does not have enough carbohydrates, it turns to protein. Each cell hoards protein in the form of amino acids, which cells can use to repair themselves, or to reproduce. When the carbohydrate supply is exhausted and an alternate source of energy is needed, the brain instructs cells to send their amino acids to the liver to be converted to glucose.

This means that anybody who is under stress for any length of time—be it biochemical, structural or emotional—is going to become protein deficient.

Only when the body is protein deficient will it turn to lipids, or fats.

While every cell in the body is capable of using fat for energy, if the need arises, the brain is not able to convert fat to glucose fast enough to keep working. It needs high-octane fuel. This is why the brain gets first dibs on all available glucose.

As discussed in the last chapter, when it comes to maintaining homeostasis, the hypothalamus pretty much runs the show. This gland responds to signals from various tissues and organs via the autonomic nervous system, which uses the sympathetic and parasympathetic controls to maintain balance. If the autonomic system wants the heart to run faster, it sends the signal through the sympathetic nervous system; if it wants the heart to run slower, it runs it through the parasympathetic nervous system.

So when the body is in a fight-or-flight situation, the sympathetic system kicks in, making the heart run faster, which increases blood flow to muscles, while reducing blood flow to organs not needed to meet the fight- or-flight challenge, in particular, the digestive organs.

Whatever the stress—emotional, chemical or structural; acute or chronic—the sympathetic response is always the same:

- Increased arterial pressure and constriction of the blood vessels, resulting in an increase in blood pressure and more blood pumped to the extremities, as opposed to the core of the body. Whether it's a person in a fight-or-flight situation, or a caregiver under chronic emotional stress, this is the sympathetic response.

- Increased blood flow to active muscles, combined with decreased blood flow to organs not needed for rapid activity. This means decreased blood flow to the digestive system, resulting in digestive symptoms and involuntary muscle contractions as the digestive organs struggle to do their jobs.

- Increased rates of cellular metabolism throughout the body. This means that the cells are consuming more nutrition and putting out more waste, which places a greater challenge on organ systems responsible for maintaining homeostasis. This is all driven by the thyroid's production of thyroxine. Under constant demand, supplies of protein, calcium and magnesium needed to produce thyroxine can run out. It's at this point that an overstressed person's metabolic rate slows down, they feel like they have no energy, and the synthetic hormone, Synthroid®, may be prescribed.

- **Increased glycolysis in muscle.** This is when the muscles convert stored glycogen to glucose to meet their own increased energy needs, which means it won't be available for the rest of the body.

- **Increased blood clotting ability.** This is why people under chronic stress are advised to take low-dose aspirin daily, to break up clots as they form.

- **Increased conversion of glycogen to glucose by the liver.** When glucose levels fall, the liver converts glycogen to glucose and releases it into the blood for transport to the brain and the reproductive system. When the body is under chronic stress, a person's energy bank account can become overdrawn and they can begin having difficulty making it through the day, both physically and mentally. The stress of continual mental activity itself is enough to bring about a body-wide energy crisis. Physiological studies conducted on Grand Master Chess players have shown that they use as much energy as a boxer fighting 10 rounds!

- **Increased conversion of cellular amino acids to glucose by the liver.** As noted earlier, when the body runs out of glucose, it turns to protein contained in body cells in the form of amino acids.

People doing mental work will run out of glucose more quickly under stress. Stress is hardest on heavy thinkers, particularly as it affects the reproductive system.

Again, all of the above apply to all manner of stress, from the immediate fight-or-flight situation to the chronic emotional stress one goes through caring for an elderly parent, or a developmentally challenged child, or the stress a young girl goes through as she approaches pubescence.

☆ Now, the only system in the human body that does respond to the stress "call to action" is the reproductive system. So when the body is stressed and down to burning fat, the last system that's going to get its share of the fat is the reproductive system, which relies on lipids for every aspect of its being, from the production of hormones that drive and regulate it to the production of eggs to perpetuate the species.

[margin note: reproductive system + lipids]

With this in mind, it makes sense that female athletes who are under extreme physical stress are known to not have periods. They're burning every drop of stored fat in their bodies. It also explains why women under a great deal of emotional stress would have a difficult time becoming pregnant, or why a young girl who is fat deficient because of chronic stress and/or a fat-deficient diet might experience a delay in her first period.

Genetics plays a key role, but without adequate lipids, there can be no menstruation.

More Information Please

If only there was more specific information for the young woman approaching her first menstrual period.

But there isn't. Nothing about when it will start or what changes it will bring with it—because everyone is different.

There is no real dependable information coming from the medical profession in terms of menstruation, let alone the child approaching her first period. The response from the medical profession has simply been to treat the symptoms with medications, as they occur.

Imagine you are a young girl approaching menarche. Though highly anticipated, no one can tell you when your period is going to start. All they know is, it starts somewhere between ages 9 and 16, though I've had patients who didn't start menstruating until they were 17.

You know it is coming because you've been prepared for it, though some women say they were never prepared for it—not by their family doctors, parents or their teachers. They just found themselves crying for no reason one day. Then the bleeding started and they couldn't figure out what was going on.

Up until that point, girls and boys were considered pretty much the same—playing in the schoolyard, making friends, participating in sports, studying, learning—all part of the great adventure of life on the Earth.

Back in my day, some girls were called "tomboys." That's a term you don't hear much anymore. I used to hear it all the time when I was growing up. My mother was a tomboy. She was a good baseball player when she was 12 years old, she told us. She used to play baseball with the boys, and she was never left off the team. She was always a good player.

When I was 11 or 12, in 1949, living in East Aurora, New York, up near Buffalo, we used to play touch football at a home in one of the nicer residential areas. The large tree-lined lawn was perfect for our games. The only condition was that we allowed the girl who lived there to play with us, while her dad and some other adults acted as referees.

I was very fast and a good pass catcher. So I wound up playing the line, opposite this man's daughter, who was bigger and stronger than I was.

Loomis, I was told, you've got to stop her. I remember having this fleeting moment thinking, "I don't want to hurt her."

Well, I got over that in a hurry. There was no stopping her. I could slow her down, but that was about it.

I remember thinking, my God, this girl is in the same grade as me and she's bigger than I am. And stronger!

My grandson is on the wrestling team, where girls wrestle with the boys. I've been to his matches. The girls are pretty strong, and while they don't necessarily push the boys around, the boys aren't able to dominate them. Heaven forbid the boy loses. I am told some boys just refused to wrestle, thus forfeiting the match.

As I said before, you don't hear the expression "tomboy" much anymore. Today, I hear women talking about their daughter as being a "girly girl."

Girls and Food

There's a lot of pressure on girls, which is why a lot of them don't eat right. They don't like to eat protein and fat because they don't want to gain weight. Again, fats are needed to make hormones. If a person doesn't eat protein and fat, they're going to wind up eating a lot of sugar for energy.

Women go through life like this.

The fact that some girls develop breasts and begin menstruating sooner than others has a lot to do with genetics.

However, it's also true that breast tissue is comprised of fat, and ovulation is not possible without lipids.

This is where young women in general come up short nutritionally, and hormonally—many do not like the taste of meat and avoid protein and fats for fear of weight gain and body image. As a father and grandfather I know there is also the issue of empathy for animals.

The person involved in strenuous exercise is going to use up their carbohydrate supply pretty quickly. Now the body has to take stored protein from cells for production of glucose, and finally the body turns to stored fat and converts that to energy. As noted, once the fat is being used for energy, it is no longer available to adequately make hormones. Consider the Female Athlete Triad, so common today, which is composed of energy deficiency, menstrual dysfunction and bone loss.

In my clinical experience 90 to 95 percent of my female patients were protein deficient.

Let's Look at Protein

Protein is essential for growth and tissue repair, especially for hair, skin, and nails. It is also essential for the formation of essential body compounds. These include hemoglobin, insulin, epinephrine and thyroxin. Dopamine, which is responsible for alertness, and the calming chemical serotonin are both protein molecules. And almost all antibodies are gamma globulin molecules.

59

Then there are the plasma proteins, which are essential in the maintenance of acid-alkaline balance, as well as regulation of water balance, transport of nutrients and cellular waste, and removal of toxic waste. Plasma proteins are also essential for maintaining calcium levels in the body, as noted in Chapter 1.

How much protein do women require? The recommended daily intake for individuals ranges from 9.1 to 13.5 grams for infants up to 12 months old; 13 to 19 grams for children ages 1 to 8; 34 to 46 grams for women ages 9 to 70; and 71 grams per day for pregnant and lactating women.

Symptoms of a protein deficiency include: increased secretions in the mouth, nose and eyes; swelling of the hands and feet, cold hands and feet, muscle cramps at night, menstrual cramps, hormonal imbalances, bleeding gums, and low tolerance for exercise.

Ringing any bells?

Protein is what separates men from women, in terms of nutrition. The lack of it in one's diet, or a failure to fully digest the protein one consumes—which is where Howell's plant enzymes come in—is a major force driving the lifelong emotional roller coaster many women experience from the day they ovulate and become a woman.

Diet plays a huge role in this emotional roller coaster, as well as other symptoms associated with menstruation, from day one.

I have seen this in my own family.

Nutrition in Other Cultures

One of my granddaughters was having problems with her period from the day it started. She was a card-carrying PETA vegetarian and wouldn't listen when her mother tried to tell her it might be her diet that was causing all the cramping, bloating, cold hands and feet, the waves of emotionality and other symptoms that came and went with each monthly cycle.

I tried talking to her, too. But she had her mind made up on this matter, until a high school trip taught her otherwise.

My granddaughter is a very bright girl and she had the opportunity to travel abroad throughout her high school years. She went to Australia one summer, and Costa Rica the next. It was during her two weeks in Costa Rica, though, that she learned about the impact that diet can have on a woman's menstrual health.

The middle-class Costa Rican family she lived with during those two weeks did not eat like middle-class families in the United States. Suddenly, my granddaughter found herself on a relatively high-protein diet, consisting of meat, beans and other high-protein foods.

When she came home, her first words to me were, "I guess you were right," because her symptoms went entirely away when she was in Costa Rica.

Her sister, who is nine years younger, is listening to her mother. We went out to breakfast on my birthday and, at her mother's suggestion, she ordered some bacon with her strawberry blintzes. She doesn't seem to be having any problems.

Generally speaking, women don't think they need as much protein as men. And while men tend to eat more protein, they only need a few grams more than women.

The bottom line: women need protein.

And this need, along with the need for calcium, becomes critical in the years leading up to menarche.

It's all about Eve becoming Eve. And you becoming you.

It's all about good nutrition, and delivering the nutrients we consume to our body's cells, which is where Howell's plant enzymes come in.

So let's move on.

CHAPTER 3

What Could Go Wrong?

The Young Adult Years

A friend once suggested that a fitting subtitle for Shakespeare's tragic tale of young, star-crossed lovers, *Romeo and Juliet,* might be, *What Could Go Wrong?*

Indeed.

Within a span of four days, Shakespeare's Juliet is courted by Count Paris, falls in love with (and secretly marries) Romeo, who, after one night of bliss with his beloved bride, is forced to flee the city because he has killed Juliet's first cousin. At that point, Juliet, all but disowned by her parents for refusing to marry the man of their choice, spends two days in a state of drug-induced unconsciousness, awakens to find herself widowed (Romeo has swallowed a potion to appear dead) and takes her own life.

All this at the tender age of 13.

Talk about stress!

Shakespeare's decision to make Juliet 13 no doubt had to do with his desire to capture her at the most innocent and emotionally vulnerable time of her life.

For today's young Juliet in her post-menarche early adult years, entering college or trying to find her way in life, stress plays a key role in her physical as well as her emotional well-being. Being a menstruating woman, she is much more susceptible to emotional stress than a man. Then there are her nutritional habits and, not least of all, which birth control option she chooses, or is chosen for her, to protect her from the ultimate life changer—the unplanned pregnancy.

All three of these potential choices will affect how she adjusts to her monthly cycle, as well as the overall quality of her life—not the least of which is her roller coaster emotions.

These days, there is also the problem of strenuous exercise, which many females are incorporating into their lives. The triad is composed of:

- Energy imbalance with or without an eating disorder
- Menstrual disturbances
- Decreased bone mineral density with or without osteoporosis.

I say *adjusts* because there are a number of years after menarche when a young woman's periods will be irregular, as her body is trying to establish itself, trying to figure out how and when to make its hormones within each cycle, and, in doing so, find its normal rhythm.

This adjustment is going to be different for every woman. Will she pitch for the softball team? Spend her free time at the library? Try out for gymnastics? The swim team? Tennis? Horseback riding? Her choices signal how she may relate to people differently in an entirely new world.

For many, the question "Am I crazy?" will resonate with each cycle.

We've seen how chronic emotional stress alone can create a glucose shortage, whereby the body is forced to burn fat for energy and come up short in lipids to produce hormones.

And so the wheel of life comes full circle.

What we're talking about in this chapter are the things that can get in the way of a woman's body finding and maintaining its normal hormonal cycle, and what can be done, nutritionally in particular, to restore normal function and help get her body and her emotional self on course to finding its natural rhythm.

Under a Wise and Brilliant Moon

We've seen what the normal cycle looks like.

We have looked at it through the lunar lens of Dr. Christine Northrup, where each phase of the moon corresponds to the rise and fall of estrogen and testosterone and the corresponding highs and lows of a woman's emotional, creative, and physical well-being, all of which will come into greater focus as we take a closer look at the cycle, particularly with regard to nutrition.

At the same time, one must bear in mind that all women are unique, and that each woman is a product of her individual genetics and her lifestyle, the combination of which has a profound influence on her individual cycle.

Recapping normal: The "normal" menstrual period is 28 days, give or take 3 days, for 65 percent of women, with an overall range of 18 to 40 days. Once a woman's menstrual pattern has been established, the variation does not normally exceed five days, with a blood loss averaging 130 milliliters, with flow generally heaviest on the second day.

Recapping abnormal: Primary or secondary amenorrhea or the absence of a menstrual cycle; erratic or irregular menstruation, whereby a woman may have three or four periods a year, or three periods close together followed by none for several months; and primary or secondary dysmenorrhea, or painful menstruation.

All this is the tip of the iceberg when one considers, as noted earlier, the hundreds of symptoms—both emotional and physiological—that have come to be associated with PMS.

Because each woman is unique, there cannot be one method of handling the common symptoms related to her "monthly blues," or period.

The same goes for figuring out which birth control pill will be best for each woman, and the pill is a major source of PMS symptoms.

Let's Talk About the Pill

The job of the birth control pill is to interfere with a woman's normal cycle in such a way as to render her infertile.

First, a closer look at the female reproductive cycle, which is divided into two phases.

The first half, or the *follicular phase,* is initiated when the anterior pituitary gland, under direction of the hypothalamus, secretes follicle-stimulating hormone (FSH) and luteinizing hormone (LH). These two hormones work together, synergistically, to regulate the reproductive processes of the body. In this first phase of the cycle, FSH stimulates the growth and recruitment of ovarian follicles in the ovary. Each follicle contains an oocyte (an immature ovum, or egg cell).

FSH and LH sharply increase during this ovulation stage.

The second half of the menstrual cycle, or luteal phase, begins after ovulation takes place, with the formation of the corpus luteum, a hormone secreting structure inside the ovary. This occurs after the mature ovum, or egg, is released from the ovary and begins its journey through the fallopian tube towards the uterus.

The luteal phase ends in either pregnancy or menstruation. If pregnancy does not occur—if an egg does not become fertilized by a sperm swimming upstream then attaching itself to the uterine wall—the corpus luteum will degenerate within a few days.

A new corpus luteum develops with each menstrual cycle.

When it's at work, the corpus luteum secretes relatively high levels of progesterone and moderate levels of estrogen in order to downgrade the production of FSH and inhibin A, which inhibits FSH production, after the egg has been released. Its secretion of estrogen inhibits further release of luteinizing hormone and follicle-stimulating hormone.

The corpus luteum is essential for establishing and maintaining pregnancy, in that its secretion of progesterone is responsible for the development and maintenance of the uterine endometrium which will nourish the developing fetus.

When the egg is not fertilized, the corpus luteum stops secreting progesterone and decays. Without progesterone, the uterine lining sloughs off and is expelled through the vagina as the menstrual period begins.

If the egg is fertilized and implantation occurs, specialized cells secrete the hormone chorionic gonadotropin (hCG), which signals the corpus luteum to continue secreting progesterone in order to maintain the thick lining of the uterus rich in blood vessels to provide nourishment to the developing embryo.

Somebody really knew what they were doing when they put all this together.

Enter the Game Changer

So where does the birth control pill come in?

The "Pill" was first approved by the FDA in the early 1960s. Its use spread rapidly, generating enormous social impact. This impact occurred because it was more effective than most previous reversible methods of contraception, giving women for the first time control over their fertility. The choice to take the birth control pill was a private one and required no special preparations at the time of sexual activity.

Claudia Goldin, an American economist, stated that this new contraceptive technology was a key player in forming women's modern economic role, in that it prolonged the age at which women first married, allowing them to become more career-oriented and invest in education. This fact is demonstrated by the sharp increase in college attendance and graduation rates for women since the advent of the Pill.

How do birth control pills work?

The whole idea behind the *combined oral contraceptive pill*, which is a combination of estrogen and progestin taken daily, is to interrupt a woman's normal cycle, and, in doing so, prevent pregnancy from occurring.

Different pills work differently in this regard.

One way the pill works is by preventing ovulation, by suppressing the release of follicle-stimulating and luteinizing hormones.

Another mechanism of action, of all progestin-containing contraceptives, is inhibiting the sperm's penetration through the cervix and uphill journey into the uterus and the fallopian tubes. It does this by decreasing the water content and increasing the viscosity of cervical mucus.

So the sperm never reaches the egg.

Hormonal contraceptives can also prevent pregnancy by altering the lining of the womb, so that a fertilized egg is not likely to become implanted.

In addition to the combined oral contraceptive pill, there is the progestin-only mini-pill, which is taken daily and does not contain estrogen, and extended-cycle pills, which contain a full complement of hormones, but are taken continuously for 12 weeks, followed by one week on an inactive pill, at which point the woman has a menstrual cycle.

Then there's the progestin-loaded birth control shot, which is given every three months, and works by preventing the ovaries from releasing eggs, and by thickening the cervical mucus, making it more difficult for the sperm to reach the egg.

The problem is, the first injection contains enough hormones—progestin, estrogen, and a little testosterone—to carry a woman for three months. When too many hormones hit the system at once, it falls on the liver to detoxify this hormonal lipid surge. This is a two-step process accomplished by two enzymes residing in the liver. One enzyme converts hormone molecules from fat soluble to water soluble, by adding an oxygen molecule, and the other enzyme quenches the resulting toxic free radical formation. When the liver becomes overworked, the result is acne, as toxins are pushed out of the body—excreted—through the skin.

This is how hormone surges during puberty result in acne, in boys as well as girls. It's not the chocolate bar. It's not the fat in the diet that causes the acne; it's the overwhelming surge of lipid-related hormones.

Further, when the woman taking the birth control shot reaches the last month, she is hormone depleted.

Because each form of hormonal birth control is designed to interfere with normal function, each will be associated with certain side effects.

A common side effect is water gain, which means the woman may require a diuretic to get rid of that excess water. This results in constipation, so now she will need a laxative.

Other side effects of hormonal birth control include: nausea, weight gain, sore or swollen breasts, spotting between periods, lighter periods, mood changes, abdominal pain, chest pain, headaches, blurred vision, and swelling or aching in the legs and thighs.

Drospirenone-containing birth control pills, like YAZ®, which, originally advertised for so-called PMSD, or PMS-associated depression, carry a risk of life-threatening blood clots. In 2012, there were more than 12,000 lawsuits against Bayer® involving YAZ® and other oral contraceptives containing drospirenone. By that time the company had already settled 1,977 such cases for $402 million.

Each different type of hormonal birth control is going to interfere with a woman's cycle differently because each woman is unique—genetically, physiologically and in terms of her lifestyle—and a woman's stress level will also be a factor. This includes all of the attending stresses that come with living on this planet. For many women finding the right pill is a hit-and-miss project.

This is the challenge facing each woman—finding the pill that works best for her, with symptoms she can live with. None of them are going to work perfectly, because they interfere with normal function.

So for each woman it comes down to which pill is better for less cramping, or which is better for less bleeding, or which is better for less water gain, or which is better for less depression, and so on.

Many patients have told me that for them it comes down to "finding the pill that makes me the least crazy."

For the health care provider, it's imperative that each woman be looked at as an individual—genetically, physiologically and in terms of her individual lifestyle. There is no one pill or medication that will work on everyone. And therein lies the problem—the puzzle wrapped in an enigma and shrouded in mystery—that all practitioners are confronted with.

And I'll say it again, when it comes to the pill, it's pretty much hit and miss.

So how does one take some of the hit and miss out of all this? By looking at each individual woman's diet, and by using nutritional strategies to restore normal function.

Women's Nutrition

Very little research has been done concerning nutritional habits of women in their early adult years. This is what led Canadian researchers to do a study of college students in 2009.

The study postulated that poor nutritional practices and increased levels of stress "are two common attributes of university life," and that they are "strongly linked to decreased health."

Indeed, by the time a young woman enters college, these two issues have already shaped who she is and what symptoms will predominate during her monthly period. Moreover, they will continue to be predominate issues as she progresses through her life. For health care providers to not understand this is to treat her as just another woman.

The study recruited 132 male and female undergraduate students who were asked to complete both lifestyle and eating behavior questionnaires. Students whose living arrangements had not changed since high school—i.e., they continued to live at home—consumed less alcohol than students who had moved away from their previous dwellings.

Not surprising, males consumed more alcohol than females.

Fast food consumption was "significantly related to lower physical activity levels and higher expenditures for food on campus," which was more common among the students who were no longer living at home and thus prone to fast food consumption. Those students living at home were more likely to pack a homemade lunch.

Consideration for healthy eating, weight control, and general wellness is of growing importance in Western society. Despite this focus on wellness, however, North Americans are on average becoming heavier, sleeping less and experiencing more stress. And weight gain has been specifically linked to undergraduate students (the infamous Freshman 15) who experience stress due to the workload of attending university.

The social pressure to fit the image of the "ideal woman" has a large impact on the way young girls and women view their bodies. Trying to live up to the images they see in popular media is difficult, if not impossible. Eating disorders are prevalent among young women of college age. Under-eating, overeating and bingeing are perhaps ways to hide their feelings, or, in the case of anorexia, restricting eating as a way of taking control of their bodies.

Food, Stress, and the Reproductive Cycle

Poor nutritional practices and increased levels of stress are two variables that will determine how a woman experiences her monthly reproductive style. And it is a woman's reproductive system that will be the significant factor that determines how she will be treated by the health care community.

> Nutrition policy and most nutrition interventions are mainly aimed at preventing birth defects and producing healthy babies. Not as much attention is paid to the individual mother's health. To that end, a woman, as a pregnant and lactating mother, may be the target but not the intended beneficiary of her health care.

Clearly, the health and nutritional status of women is important for the survival and healthy development of her children, but there is a lot more to a woman than just reproduction.

A better approach might be to put a greater focus on female health and nutrition throughout a woman's life cycle, as opposed to the traditional concerns with maternal nutrition during pregnancy and lactation.

My own mother and grandmother, both of whom were registered nurses, taught me that both the woman and the man must prepare their bodies well in advance of attempting to produce a baby.

This is the teaching that was bred into me.

What this comes down to is taking a life-cycle approach to both the analysis of nutritional problems and the choice of interventions that emphasize that nutritional status, which, unlike disease, is cumulative over time and not an isolated incident.

The lifestyle approach highlights the centrality of nutrition in maintaining women's health.

About Malnutrition

Poor nutrition often starts in utero, before a child is born, and extends, particularly for girls and women, through their life cycle. It also spans generations. Malnutrition that occurs during childhood, adolescence, and pregnancy has an additive negative impact on the birth weight of future babies.

Malnutrition has major consequences for women, affecting their health, productivity, and overall quality of life. It may also affect their chances of survival. Of the four main causes of maternal death in childbirth, three—hemorrhage, infection, and obstructed labor—are related directly or indirectly to nutrition.

When it comes to pregnancy, which we will be discussing in the next chapter, pre-pregnancy weight, pregnancy weight gain, and iron status are critical indicators of pregnancy outcomes for both the mother and the newborn. And iron deficiency is directly related to protein metabolism, and only protein metabolism! It begins and ends with adequate protein ingestion and digestion. This is something that many women don't realize.

"I don't like protein," women have said to me, referring primarily to meat. "It doesn't make me feel good."

This is the direct result of poor digestion, inadequate stomach acid and poor gallbladder function, all of which can be overcome with the addition of plant enzyme supplementation specific to each woman's diet and individual needs.

Anemia related to inadequate protein ingestion and digestion is pervasive among young women. In my own clinical experience, it follows them throughout their lives.

The most common symptoms of anemia include general fatigue and compromised immune function.

Another contributing factor to protein deficiency in menstruating women is the shedding of the uterine lining when pregnancy does not occur—when no fertilized egg attaches to the wall of the uterus. The endometrium and supporting tissues require a substantial amount of protein to be formed. When this lining is shed, during menstruation, a lot of protein leaves the body. If the woman is already protein deficient because of inadequate protein in her diet and/or inadequate digestion, the impact of the protein loss during the luteal phase and menstruation becomes even greater.

Adolescent girls are particularly vulnerable to the effects of malnutrition. Underweight adolescent girls may not finish growing before their first pregnancy. Still-growing adolescents are likely to give birth to a smaller baby than a mature woman of the same nutritional status, due to poorer placental function and competition for nutrients between the growing mother and the growing fetus.

> **It has been my clinical experience that most of my female patients have been protein deficient, and this is the root cause of many of their health challenges, certainly non-disease-related menstrual problems.**

There are four separate and distinct dietary patterns involved in PMS, which we will discuss shortly. The successful treatment of this problem must be aimed at discovering who it is we are treating, with regard to each individual woman's nutritional status, as opposed to just blocking symptoms with medications.

Key in this discussion is understanding the functions of dietary protein:

1. **Protein is essential for growth and tissue repair.** It is not a stretch to say that growth is only possible when there is an adequate supply of protein over and above the amount needed for maintenance and repair of tissue. Females need to know that hair, skin, and nails require larger amounts of sulfur-containing protein found in animal protein and dark leafy greens.

2. **Formation of essential body compounds.** Hormones such as insulin, adrenaline, and thyroxine are all proteins, along with estrogen and progesterone, of course. Hemoglobin and almost all of the factors involved in blood clotting are proteins. The photoreceptors in the eye that are responsible for vision are proteins. The neurotransmitters dopamine (alertness chemical) and serotonin (calming chemical) are proteins. During any protein-deficiency state, the production of certain of these protein compounds receive priority over other less important protein functions.

3. **Antibodies for immune function are proteins.** In impoverished Third World countries, protein deficiency accounts for a large amount of infant mortality among malnourished children because specific antibodies against infection cannot be formed.

4. **Regulation of water balance.** The accumulation of fluid in the tissues is an early warning sign of protein deficiency, thus giving the tissues a soft, spongy, bloated appearance (edema).

My mentioning that most of my female patients have been protein deficient may be met with some objection from health care providers who routinely examine blood test results and find no signs of protein deficiency.

 This is a widespread misconception! It is uncommon among otherwise healthy females to have low amounts of protein on routine blood tests when they are protein deficient. The reason for this is that plasma proteins are essential in maintaining homeostasis in the blood and the extracellular fluids, for the transport of nutrients in the blood and waste to be removed from the body. And when more protein is required in the blood to maintain normal function it moves amino acids out of the cell where they would have been used for growth and repair.

As noted earlier, half the calcium in the blood is bound to plasma proteins. The other half is free floating to prevent muscle (menstrual) cramps, among other things. This ratio never changes. When the protein levels drop in the blood, calcium will show up in urine tests. It is uncommon for otherwise healthy females to have low amounts of plasma proteins on routine blood tests.

For a protein deficiency to actually show up in the blood, the person must be seriously ill.

On the other side of the coin, calcium has homeostatic relationships with other molecules, such as phosphorus, potassium and magnesium, among others. These relationships are also disturbed when available calcium is lowered for any length of time. Looking for excessive amounts of calcium being discarded in the urine (in relation to pH) was routine training during my chiropractic education, and I used it throughout my career in treating patients, especially those with menstrual problems.

What follows are the four basic *diet-related reproductive syndromes* I found I could quickly identify in a patient's case history and use to put together a treatment strategy to restore normal function. Many women reading this book will no doubt see their own reproductive selves in the descriptions of these syndromes, and the composite cases I have created to illustrate these syndromes.

These are the four faces of PMS as they appear in the young Juliet as she enters the world and as she will make her way through life.

Please remember that medical studies, the latest in 2012, found over 100 symptoms associated with PMS and so dividing them into four classes is for convenience only.

PMS-A: The High Anxiety, Irritable Type

As noted earlier, 80 percent of women with PMS have symptoms characteristic of this group. These symptoms are predominantly anxiety-related, and are driven by excess estrogen, a central nervous system stimulant.-Or, high estrogen levels may actually be related to a deficiency in progesterone, resulting in a high estrogen-to-progesterone ratio—not enough progesterone to quiet things down.

Symptoms of anxiety may also be the result of body's inability to break down estrogen, due to poor liver function or vitamin B deficiency.

Then there's calcium. One of the cardinal signs of a calcium deficiency is irritability progressing slowly to minor numbness or tingling of the fingers, muscle (menstrual) cramps, lethargy and poor appetite.

This reflects the very difficult situation of low total calcium, which causes irritability and anxiety, accompanied by low ionized calcium, which is needed to prevent cramping, combined with poor protein digestion.

Remember: as protein levels go down, so do calcium levels.

Vitamin D supplementation may help improve calcium levels, but it does not address protein deficiency, and if you don't have the protein to hold the calcium, it won't do any good.

So here's Anne. She's past menarche, in college or finding her way in the workplace, and by this time in her young life, her periods are probably regular, or close to it.

And she's protein deficient, because she's not consuming enough protein, and/or not digesting what she is consuming, besides losing a substantial amount of protein every time she cycles, as her body uses protein to build up her uterine wall in anticipation of a pregnancy, and sheds it when there is no pregnancy to support.

And because she's protein deficient, she's also going to become calcium deficient. 50 percent of calcium in the blood is bound to protein, and when protein goes down, calcium goes down and she becomes anxious and irritable, along with the previously mentioned symptoms of calcium deficiency.

Why is she not consuming protein? She may be a vegetarian, or not eating meat for ethical reasons, or she may avoid meat for religious reasons, or she may be avoiding protein simply because she doesn't feel good after she eats a high-protein meal, which means she's not digesting it properly.

Further, she has high estrogen production, which drives her anxiety and puts an added burden on her liver, so she probably has acne.

How does one go about helping this young woman?

The pharmaceutical approach would be to find the right birth control for her, but again, this is hit and miss. Remember, all women are different.

A better approach would be to figure out what her body is missing in terms of nutrition and give it the nutrition it needs to maintain normalcy.

I did this for years, with great success, observing symptoms, looking for involuntary muscle contractions to discover which organs are struggling, and by using blood tests and urinalysis to figure out where our friend Anne is nutritionally deficient.

In Anne's Type A case, we want to improve her protein intake a little—we've only got to get her up to about 43 or 44 grams of protein a day. And we have to make sure she digests it, which means giving her a supplemental plant enzyme formula with an emphasis on protease.

We would also have to supplement some calcium, and even a little vitamin D, if we think she's having trouble absorbing calcium.

> One thing to remember, these women are inevitably deficient in hydrochloric acid—i.e., stomach acid. It has to do with the protein deficiency, but it also results in problems digesting fat. You need hydrochloric acid to convert pepsinogen into pepsin, which digests protein in the stomach. The other side of the coin is that it is hydrochloric acid that thins the bile so it can flow and do its job emulsifying dietary fat so that the fat can be digested.

Without hydrochloric acid, the bile becomes sluggish and you don't emulsify the fat adequately. If not emulsified, the fat combines with any calcium in the diet, making it insoluble and eliminating it in the stool.

Hence, our young Anne is both protein and lipid deficient, and by association calcium deficient.

The key to treating all this are plant enzymes—with the emphasis on protease to make sure she digests the protein she's now eating, and lipase, to help digest fats. Add to this a small amount of calcium, and vitamin D to help her absorb the calcium.

It's the physical examination that charts the course. Do I have to focus on just protein, or do I have to focus on protein and fat? That's where the clinical judgment comes in.

The five women discussed in Chapter 1 were all Type A. After those breakthrough cases, word got around and I was overwhelmed with new patients, women coming to me with PMS. And for the first time, I no longer dreaded treating them. I actually looked forward to their arrival at my door.

CHAPTER 3—What Could Go Wrong?: *The Young Adult Years*

Because I had finally found some answers, and they were so motivated and so grateful for the relief I was able to give them.

PMS-C: The Type A Personality Sugar Bear

Approximately 40 percent of women with PMS symptoms present with problems related to carbohydrate cravings. This is often due to increased responsiveness to insulin. The "Sugar Bear" consumes excessive amounts of simple sugar. She also may consume so-called sugar substitutes (artificial sweeteners), which the body cannot digest and therefore provide zero calories.

Foremost on the list of this young woman's problems is that refined sugars that are absorbed into the body necessitate the use of important alkaline minerals like potassium and magnesium, and even sodium, along with B vitamins, to metabolize them, thereby reducing the availability of these key minerals and vitamins for more important functions. All this results in stress to the body, particularly the respiratory system, and the kidneys, setting off the fight-or-flight cascade, and depleting stored energy sources for important body functions.

These young women are susceptible to adrenal exhaustion because of continued sympathetic stimulation, and because of alkaline mineral deficiency. Hence they don't have a lot of lasting energy.

They just don't have the adrenaline to keep them going.

Meanwhile, all this stress causes constriction of the blood vessels that serve the body's organs, particularly the kidneys. Thus, the kidneys' ability to clean the blood is diminished, resulting in increased incidence of allergies, as well as back pain due to involuntary muscle contractions emanating from the stressed kidneys.

Back pain and allergies are very often the symptoms that will drive Sugar Bears into the doctor's office, because their kidneys aren't cleaning their blood adequately.

There's no one symptom to isolate here. These are packages of symptoms.

So what does our young Sugar Bear look like?

Again, she may be a young adult, away from home for the first time, in college or finding her way in the workplace. More often than not, she's unmarried and not in a committed relationship.

This is important, because there's a lot of stress-related issues for a female in this age group, as she tries to find her place in the world, dating, taking the Pill or not taking the Pill, forever mindful of the risk of pregnancy while she looks for commitment in a relationship.

It's a perfect storm, sort of.

Most young vegetarians are in reality *"pastatarians", not all,* but most young vegetarians are: They don't want to eat meat, so they mix vegetables in with their pasta and call themselves vegetarians.

Once consumed, however, pasta quickly breaks down to simple sugar, which is then converted to fat.

So there's your Sugar Bear, constantly craving sugar. She's a Type A personality with very little patience, subject to irritability, and road rage. And she's ambitious.

It's a package deal. With excessive sugar consumption, the body uses up important alkaline minerals to metabolize these sugars, resulting in constipation, irritability and even the loss of the ability to think clearly.

Magnesium deficiency in itself is often related to the emotional roller coaster phenomenon.

The Sugar Bear craves sugar. Any time you're taking in sugar, you're going to want more.

The key to treating this young woman, I soon realized, started with making her aware that it was her sugar consumption that was driving her symptoms.

I then explained to her that in order to turn off her sugar cravings, I had to improve her sugar digestion, by giving her a pre-digestive enzyme supplement. If I did that, I explained, and you don't change your diet, you're going to gain weight.

Offering the truth about possible weight gain, which *no one* ever wants to happen, will usually result in a positive outcome. You might say, it worked like a charm!

While the plant enzyme supplement I concocted was primarily formulated to digest sugar, protease was also a key ingredient, as was lipase, *because most women are protein deficient* because—and this is key—at the very bottom of every Sugar Bear's nutritional being is fat deficiency stemming from her inability to adequately digest fat.

In a word, she wasn't digesting fat, so her body was converting incoming sugar to fat and storing it. This is the woman who is going to grow up to be a member of the 4F club, *female, forty, fat and fertile*. That is an unfortunate memory key taught to many clinicians of my generation.

However, within two weeks of her being off sugar, with the pre-digestive enzymes ensuring that her body was digesting the nutrients she was taking in, her sugar cravings were gone and she didn't have to worry about gaining weight.

And as the sugar disappeared from her diet, so did her depletion of alkaline minerals and all the rest.

From then on, whenever I had a patient who was on birth control pills and had carbohydrate cravings, I knew exactly what to do.

So the key in treating the Sugar Bear with PMS is threefold. First is getting them to cut down on their sugar consumption, including pasta, which will then reduce their craving for sugar. Then provide them with alkaline minerals to relieve their adrenal exhaustion and improve their kidney function. And finally, give them a plant enzyme supplement that includes sucrase, maltase and lactase to improve sugar digestion, as well as a protease to improve protein digestion, and finally a lipase to improve their digestion of fat.

Plant enzyme supplementation is the key. Like everyone else, the Sugar Bear needs to be able to digest what she eats.

PMS-H: The Slow Metabolism Type

This group of symptoms affects about 60 percent of women with PMS.

Signs and symptoms are predominantly bloating and edema, increased levels of ACTH (the stress hormone) and increased aldosterone secretion to preserve water and salt by the kidneys.

In other words, they're holding water, and it's leaking out into the tissues, so they have edema.

These women are under chronic stress. As a result they suffer from what appears to be **HYPOTHYROIDISM**—their thyroid gland is overworked and unable to produce enough thyroxin to keep them going.

So there's your slow metabolism.

Their calcium levels may be adequate enough to prevent their muscle cramping from progressing to numbness and tingling. But there is inadequate stomach acid, and either poor protein ingestion or digestion, along with biliary stress, even if their gallbladder has been removed. This is because the bile is coming from the liver. The gallbladder just stores it.

It's protein digestion that creates acidity, and the biliary distress is due to the lack of stomach acid needed to thin bile out and get it flowing.

This young woman needs supplemental plant enzymes to enhance protein and fat digestion, heavy ended on lipase, as well as fatty acids, and calcium and magnesium, all of this aimed at nutritionally supporting her thyroid gland and improving her metabolic rate.

Such a regimen can take the hit and miss out of PMS treatment.

It's all about giving the body what it needs, and treating each woman as an individual, with individual needs. There's no magic bullet.

PMS-D: The ANTACID or Proton Pump Inhibitor User

On the matter of what has been termed **PMS-D**, only about five percent of PMS sufferers are primarily affected by depression related to excessive progesterone, a central nervous system depressant. Nutritional supplementation is of little help in this situation. And clearly, treatment of clinical depression is beyond my expertise.

Nevertheless, my experience has been that having the symptoms associated with PMS following every ovulation in each menstrual cycle can be stressful if not debilitating.

Therefore I was motivated to help as much as possible. In that regard, there is a digestive syndrome intimately related to a large part of the female population. Recall that stress irritates the lining of the stomach and is responsible for the symptoms of what has been called excess stomach acid—i.e., heartburn, etc.

However—and here's the rub—it is impossible for the body to make excess stomach acid!

The term itself is a misnomer.

The symptoms of heartburn do not come from excess stomach acid. Rather, this burning sensation occurs when stomach acid irritates the protective mucosal lining of the stomach wall. So preventing or reducing the formation of stomach acid with a proton pump inhibitor can be a good thing—for a limited time, to give the mucosal lining time to heal.

The problem is, proton pump inhibitors have become the treatment of choice for any and all digestive issues.

So here's our young Juliet, who comes to her doctor seeking birth control, and who explains she has digestive problems. Without running any tests, he puts her on a proton pump inhibitor to relieve her digestive symptoms. He doesn't know whether her symptoms are related to the stomach, the biliary system, the pancreas or sugar digestion.

The symptoms are often so vague that they defy specific diagnosis. Better to just turn off the stomach acid.

However, using proton pump inhibitors long term has a downside—stomach acid is needed to convert pepsinogen into pepsin, which is the first step in protein digestion!

Further, blocking protein digestion seriously disturbs the relationship between protein and calcium, and even phosphorus! This is what bone is made of—protein, calcium and phosphorous. This is why people who are on long-term proton pump inhibitors have spontaneous fractures of the long bones, like the femur.

What causes the mucosal lining of the stomach to become thin and irritated in the first place is stress. Any time a person is under stress, the mucosal lining becomes inflamed; it turns red! It is this stress reaction on the part of the stomach lining that is responsible for the so-called symptoms of excess stomach acid.

Whenever a woman with PMS came to me with digestive symptoms who was taking a proton pump inhibitor, the first thing I would do is get her off the proton pump inhibitor and find out what she was having trouble digesting—protein, carbohydrates, fats, etc.—and give her the plant enzymes to improve her digestion.

I would also give her plant enzymes and mucilaginous herbs STM aimed at nourishing the stomach lining, such as marshmallow root, okra, and slippery elm—things that produce mucilage when you digest them.

Of course, she's going to be protein deficient. So a protein supplement would be in order, either an herbal form or things like eggs, cheese or yeast. Cheese and bratwurst are a favorite in Wisconsin where I live.

Before all of this, however, is the need to identify and reduce her stress. Is it structural, emotional or visceral? Is it her lifestyle? University classes? Her family? Or even her new business or job or money problems? Is it student loans? Or the IRS? Whatever it is, it has to be identified and she has to do something about it.

A Final Word About Depression

PMS-D has been used as a marketing tool by the pharmaceutical industry for certain birth control pills allegedly aimed at helping people with PMS-related depression. European medical societies have rejected this from the beginning. Why? Because there is no separate group of PMS sufferers who are more susceptible to depression.

Quite simply, when any person suffers from PMS symptoms long enough, they are going to become depressed. Depression is the end result of the degenerative process.

It all comes down to stress.

Hans Selye had figured it out, right down to the nutritional fix.

These are the faces of PMS, as they apply to all women entering womanhood—from the Mother of us all, to Shakespeare's Juliet, and to the modern woman.

CHAPTER 4

A Balancing Act

From Prevention to Pregnancy

During the course of the last two chapters we watched as our young Juliet made her way to womanhood, from puberty to her first menstrual period. We watched her struggle with the hormonal ups and downs that came in waves as her newly fertile body began seeking its normal hormonal rhythm.

We saw her doing her best to live with her PMS symptoms, unaware of underlying nutritional deficiencies that contributed to these strange new symptoms. These protein, lipid and carbohydrate deficiencies resulted from inadequate ingestion or digestion of nutrients, and from the long-term use of proton pump inhibitors.

Then came the task of figuring out which hormonal birth control option was best for her—the one with the fewest side effects, the one that made her "the least crazy"—to prevent an unwanted pregnancy as she made her way into the world.

Over the years, the Pill has given women more options for planning their lives. It has enabled women to take control of their reproductive timeline, to become educated, to marry or not marry, to enter professions and put off having children into their middle or late 30s, even their 40s.

And yet, all this comes at a price. Whatever type of birth control a woman has chosen, its job is to prevent pregnancy. In the case of the Pill, it does this by interrupting normal function, primarily by regulating estrogen and progesterone secretion. Unfortunately, the return of normal function and fertility after a woman stops taking the Pill is not necessarily a switch-off, switch-on situation. She can go months or longer before becoming pregnant.

Some women are never able to restore normal reproductive function.

Looking back, our young Juliet wasn't in balance before she began taking the Pill, with the hormonal surges that came with menarche, in the midst of dietary deficiencies. Now all of this is suddenly compounded by interrupting her already unbalanced reproductive cycle with the hormone-manipulating, birth control pill.

Is it any wonder that her body might take time to find its way back to hormonal normalcy after years on the birth control pill? Considerable changes must take place. Often, these changes never happen.

Infertility has become a big business in the United States during the last decade, as many women in their thirties and forties who delayed pregnancy are unable to conceive. According to Western medicine, a woman is said to be infertile if conception has not occurred after 12 months of trying to conceive, although in some cases conception could take up to two or three years.

CHAPTER 4—A Balancing Act: *From Prevention to Pregnancy*

In my own practice, the subject of infertility usually came up when a woman was using the body temperature method for determining when she ovulated, when her chance of becoming pregnant was at its highest.

Basal body temperature (BBT) is the lowest body temperature that is recorded immediately after awakening and before any physical activity has been undertaken. In women, ovulation causes an increase of one-half to one degree Fahrenheit. Thus, monitoring of BBT is one way of estimating the day of ovulation.

It's important to note that BBT only shows when ovulation has occurred and cannot be used to predict ovulation.

This is usually the first strategy a woman follows when she is having difficulty becoming pregnant. If she can time intercourse with this rise in body temperature, she increases her odds of becoming pregnant.

There are so many factors contributing to infertility. There's the woman's egg supply, which is at its peak when a fetus is at 14 weeks of development. It is at this point during embryonic development that all of the eggs a female has for her lifetime have developed. Common sense tells us that by the time a woman is age 40, those eggs may not have the vitality they had 20 years earlier. Further, there will be fewer eggs, and due to their age, the chance of them being damaged has increased, making conception a bit more difficult. Instances of birth defects are greater for a woman conceiving at age 40 versus age 20.

There are many clinical causes for infertility, such as environmental toxins, poor nutrition, scarring of the fallopian tubes due to endometriosis, stress and low/immature sperm count. Low sperm count has been attributed to wearing tight underwear, which can make the testes too hot. The testes need to be two degrees cooler than the rest of the body. A simple change to boxer shorts can increase a man's sperm count.

Depending on the source consulted, the percentages attributing infertility to the male versus female varies from 40 percent male, 60 percent female, to 40 percent male, 40 percent female and 20 percent unknown. The importance of these statistics is that infertility is not solely a woman's problem as many women consciously or subconsciously believe.

Infertility has also been attributed to related emotional issues resulting in chronic stress which, as we have seen, can contribute to nutritional deficiencies. Many times when the couple relaxes and lets Nature take over, pregnancy occurs.

What this all comes down to is that conception is a *miracle* that can be taken for granted until it becomes difficult to achieve.

When infertility persists, couples will often resort to drastic and costly measures. And yet, such actions may not be necessary.

One of the most rewarding cases ever to come my way was a woman—a physician—who had failed to become pregnant despite four years of trying everything under the sun.

After a year of trying to conceive naturally, she and her husband were both medically evaluated. The first course of action was the surgical treatment of her husband to remove a varicocele (an abnormal enlargement of the venous plexus, a congregation of veins in the scrotum) and a spermatocele (a retention cyst of the tubule in the testes).

After months of waiting and still no pregnancy, the couple tried intrauterine insemination (IUI), which involves artificial introduction of the sperm into the uterus, combined with fertility drugs.

Again, no luck.

The next step to consider was in vitro fertilization (IVF), which involves close monitoring and stimulating of the woman's ovulatory process, removing the ovum, or egg, from the ovaries, and exposing them to sperm in a fluid medium in the laboratory. The fertilized egg is then cultured for two to six days in a growth medium before being implanted in the woman's uterus.

But why should the woman go through with such an expensive and perhaps "scary" procedure, when the doctors reviewing all of her tests kept saying that they could find nothing wrong physiologically with her?

Why do it? It made no sense.

She continued searching. She tried various holistic treatments, like acupuncture, chiropractic, herbs, homeopathy, naturopathy, and yoga therapy to reduce stress. This was a particularly challenging time in her life. Besides obsessing over her inability to become pregnant, she was also taking various supplements, adjusting to dietary changes, and dedicating herself to prayer.

Again, no luck. She just couldn't conceive.

By the time she came to me, my job was easier because she was already working on stress reduction, which had been contributing to her inability to conceive.

The reason all the heroic medical treatments she and her husband had undergone weren't working, I explained to her, was in all likelihood because her body was not yet ready to accept a baby. What we were going to do was go back to Nature and restore normal function, and we were going to do it with nutrition. If all went well, I figured, it would take 60 to 90 days to get her pregnant.

So we began taking the steps dictated by her body.

We started out making specific structural corrections, restoring normal pelvic alignment, combined with specific nutritional support—i.e., lipid metabolism to nourish the tissues involved.

Then came dietary changes—adding adequate amounts of protein and reducing starches and simple carbohydrates, and avoiding oils at mealtime to keep her food uncoated and readily digestible.

Fortunately I had a very compliant patient.

Third, digestion had to be improved via plant enzyme supplementation, in particular to improve stomach and biliary functions. I gave her a balanced formula, containing protease, amylase, cellulase and lipase, with an emphasis on the lipase to nourish lipid metabolism, and thus energize the hormonal system.

With improved nutrient utilization, Mother Nature did the rest.

It's amazing what the human body can do when it functions normally. The final nutritional adjustments were made in January and she was pregnant in February. She gave birth to a healthy baby boy in November. Her second son was born 18 months later.

Every so often I get pictures of two of the best-looking healthy boys you can imagine.

The point is this. If a woman's uterine wall, which is made up of protein, is not adequately prepared to receive the fertilized egg, or if her body is not producing the necessary hormones because of nutritional deficiencies, or because it's been thrown off by birth control pills, she's not going to be able to get pregnant, regardless of what medical procedures are performed. An implanted embryo is not going to survive if the uterine wall is not able to support it.

With this in mind, it made sense to me, once pathology had been ruled out as the cause of infertility, to take the nutritional approach before any heroic efforts.

> **Because infertility is not a disease, any more than PMS is a disease. They are both evidence of a lack of normal function, which the body will restore if it has the nutrition to do so. It's all about restoring normal function.**

Whether you're talking about relieving PMS symptoms or getting pregnant, the key is providing the body with the nutrition it needs and the means of digesting those nutritious foods so that the body can function the way it was intended to.

This is where it all comes together—in nutrition.

Nutrition & Pregnancy: Taking a Closer Look

So let's take a closer look at nutrition as it relates to pregnancy, starting with what we've learned about nutrition and PMS. We have seen the four types of PMS in progress.

We have seen how they can impact a young woman's physical as well as her emotional well-being as she makes her way in the world. We have also seen how each of these **four types of PMS** is uniquely tied to nutrition. Taking this one step further, the same nutritional factors tied to the four types of PMS will also impact a young woman's reproductive abilities if she decides to become a mother.

For example, the protein deficiency that is associated with the **high anxiety PMS-A type** compromises a woman's reproductive abilities because it is protein that is used to build up the uterine wall that will nourish the fetus through its development.

> This is of critical importance and I believe often completely overlooked when charting a course of dietary change and nutritional supplementation in cases of premenstrual syndrome, infertility and planning for pregnancy.

Consider the following clinical observations I made during my years of practice:

1. The vast majority of my female patients in their reproductive years were protein deficient.

2. A review of protein metabolism tells us that about 50 percent of the calcium in the blood is attached to and transported by protein. The other half is not attached to protein and is used by the body for many purposes, the best known perhaps is to prevent

CHAPTER 4—A Balancing Act: From Prevention to Pregnancy

[Margin note: Iron, HCl, Vit C]

muscle cramps. When more protein is being used for growth and tissue repair, as in thickening the uterine wall following ovulation, or during pregnancy when a placenta must be created, there is a drop in protein available to transport calcium and prevent muscle cramps. That means levels of irritability a woman experiences may increase.

3. Young women are taught that their monthly period can create an iron deficiency. A review of iron metabolism tells us that adequate stomach acid and vitamin C are needed to prepare iron to be absorbed and stored by a protein molecule (ferritin). Iron can then be attached to another protein molecule for transport through the blood and bound to yet another protein molecule (hemoglobin) inside the red blood cells. Yes, menstruation can lead to iron deficiency, but there is a lot of protein also being lost in menstrual blood. The sloughing off and discharge of the thickened uterine wall adds substantially to loss of protein that must be replaced every month!

4. There is another point that must be reiterated here. The flow of acid coming out of the stomach stimulates the flow of bile for the degreasing (emulsification) of fats. This is necessary to allow enzymes from the pancreas access to penetrate and break down the contents of the diet. Enzymes do not penetrate fats well. If the woman is deficient in stomach acid, she will struggle digesting fats that are needed for adequate hormone production necessary for pregnancy.

99

Besides calcium deficiency, protein deficiency is also associated with anemia, since hemoglobin is actually a small amount of iron attached to a very large protein molecule.

And a woman who is protein deficient will inevitably be deficient in hydrochloric acid, which, as noted, thins out bile to render fat digestible by the body's enzymes. When a woman is fat deficient, hormone production can become impaired, as well as other aspects of her ability to reproduce.

The PMS-C Sugar Bear craves carbohydrates because she doesn't digest fat well and her body needs energy. So she binges on sugar, or pasta, which quickly breaks down to simple sugar, and what is not needed for energy is stored as fat. The breakdown of simple sugars depletes the body of critical alkaline minerals. Ms. Sugar Bear is more likely to gain a lot of weight during pregnancy, and she is more susceptible to postpartum depression. And because she is also frequently protein deficient, her ability to build up her uterine wall will be compromised, and she will be hydrochloric acid deficient, which continues to impair fat digestion.

The primary nutritional problem confronting the **PMS-H type is fat digestion**. We have already outlined the cascade of nutritional problems she faces.

1. Protein deficiency

2. Stomach acid deficiency

3. Thickened bile flow (or perhaps her gallbladder has already been removed)

4. Fatty acid deficiency (accompanying inadequate or inappropriate reproductive hormone production)

5. In addition to digestive and reproductive symptoms, problems occur with her skin, hair, and nails

Again, the primary nutritional problem confronting the **PMS-H type is fat digestion**, due to hydrochloric acid deficiency leading to biliary/gallbladder problems. If a woman wants to become pregnant, the last thing she wants is to be fat deficient.

As discussed earlier, **when it comes to homeostasis, protein is king. When it comes to reproduction, fat rules.** Lipids stimulate the production of follicle-stimulating hormones (FSH), luteinizing hormone (LH) and lactogenic (LTH) hormone (prolactin), making it possible for a woman to become pregnant, carry the baby to term, induce labor, and lactate, so she can feed her baby.

All of this is dependent on adequate lipid ingestion and digestion.

Finally, there's PMS-D, which brings us to women who are taking proton pump inhibitors, H2 blockers, or antacids, all of which either block or retard the production of hydrochloric acid. When you shut down stomach acid production, you shut down or retard the important initial step in protein digestion that occurs in the stomach. Without stomach acid, bile remains thick and does not flow, and fats are not emulsified and cannot be penetrated by the body's digestive enzymes. The body is thus incapable of digesting fats, and the woman must now turn to sugar for energy.

It's a domino effect, with a lot of overlap between the different types of PMS with regard to nutritional deficiencies, resulting symptoms, and the impact these deficiencies have on a woman's ability to reproduce.

> We have witnessed the step-by-step cascade of physiological events that cause symptoms associated with a woman's reproductive monthly cycle. The good news is, if the health care provider can figure out which nutritional profile fits each individual woman and make the necessary dietary changes, and supplement the indicated plant enzymes to assist in pre-digestion, the woman will be better able to prepare her body to achieve a normal, healthy pregnancy and deliver a healthy baby. **Once again, give the body what it needs.**

This becomes even more apparent when we look at nutrition as it applies to the five stages of pregnancy.

THE FIVE STAGES OF PREGNANCY:
From an Article for Health Care Providers

Note: Here's part of an article I wrote for providers on the stages of pregnancy. As a reader, you'll notice my language is more scientific, but it's valuable for you to know.

Question: Why is it that the United States spends more money on health care than any country in the world, and yet it only ranks 34th in lowest infant mortality rate? These incongruent statistics could be attributed to the fact that U.S. health care dollars seem to be aimed at fixing problems rather than preventing them.

Pregnancy-related nutrition is a vital part of child development. In order to facilitate healthy development, both parents need to be in a state of optimal health.

Current pregnancy advice dictates that a woman should improve her diet and avoid such things as alcohol and cigarettes for the sake of her baby's health. What is not fully appreciated or understood is that some of the most important fetal development occurs during the first three weeks of pregnancy. Just 18 days after conception, the baby's heart begins to beat and life begins to take shape. The neural tube, out of which will grow the brain and the spinal chord, also begins to develop during the third week.

Unfortunately, many women do not even know that they are pregnant at this time. For this reason, potential mothers must include preconception as an important stage in planning for a baby as well as the residual effects of postpartum lactation and depression.

With this in mind, we can separate pregnancy-related nutrition into five stages: *Preparing for Conception, the First Trimester, the Second Trimester,* the *Third Trimester,* and lastly *Postpartum.* By focusing on the five nutritional stages of pregnancy, health care providers can help their patients be fully prepared for the birth of a healthy child.

STAGE ONE:
PREPARING FOR CONCEPTION

A lot of work is involved when starting a family. But before future parents stock up on diapers and baby bottles it is important that they are in an optimum state of health in order to conceive a child.

Parents-to-be should adhere to the following guidelines three months prior to the attempt at conception:

- Get plenty of sleep, at least seven to eight hours per night. If more sleep is not possible, rest.
- Drink lots of water; it is necessary to cleanse the body.
- Exercise as much as possible. At the very least go for walks.
- Stop drinking alcohol and smoking.
- Eat a healthy and balanced diet.

Even if you believe that you are eating well you may still have occasional cravings. Cravings are an indication of nutritional problems that should be addressed immediately.

It is important to recognize that even individuals who feel that they consume healthy, balanced diets may develop vitamin and mineral deficiencies. *The 1988 Surgeon General Report on Health and Nutrition* emphatically states that the overwhelming problem in nutrition is nutrient excess rather than deficiency. Thus, the problem must stem from nutrient assimilation, which begins with digestion and absorption.

Preconception and Prenatal Nutrition

"Prenatal" means prior to birth, not prior to conception. This term is often misused and it is important to understand its true meaning when speaking in terms of nutrition. If possible, prenatal nutrition should begin several months prior to conception to prepare the bodies of both parents for a baby.

A nutrient deficiency in either parent will influence child development before and after the birth. Some of the most important fetal development occurs within the first month of pregnancy. If a woman has a deficiency before she becomes pregnant and does not receive nutritional support (prenatal vitamins) until roughly another month after conception, it will be difficult, if not impossible, to play catch up.

Good prenatal nutrition cannot be confined to a bottle labeled, "prenatal multiple vitamin and mineral supplement." Many prenatal vitamin and mineral products contain ingredients of the cheapest quality that can be legally sold. These poor quality supplements may create a feeling of nausea in expectant mothers because they are unable to properly digest or assimilate the products.

The standard prenatal recommendation is to supplement folic acid for the prevention of neural tube defects in the baby. However, as noted, the neural tube develops within the first three weeks of pregnancy, and many mothers-to-be do not even know that they are pregnant at this time.

More emphasis should be placed on the importance of lipid digestion and assimilation for both males and females in order to prepare for the conception and development of a fetus. Improved fatty acid digestion and correction of any fatty acid deficiency is paramount in ensuring a healthy pregnancy and delivery.

Fatty Acids

Fatty acids are the "problem" with problem pregnancies. They control the ability to impregnate, conceive, prevent spontaneous abortion, induce labor appropriately, and commence lactation. However, in this day of great technological research and advances such as artificial insemination, fertility pills, and in-vitro fertilization, essential nutrients—i.e., fatty acids—have taken a backseat to the latest and greatest pharmaceutical development.

> **For the record:**
>
> *Linoleic acid*, an 18-carbon fatty acid with two double bonds, promotes growth and heals dermatitis. It cannot be produced by the body and therefore must be included in the diet. It can be found in vegetable and seed oils such as safflower, sunflower, corn, soybean, cottonseed, sesame, and peanut. Linoleic acid is a polyunsaturated omega-6 fatty acid.
>
> *Arachidonic acid* is a 20-carbon polyunsaturated fatty acid with four double bonds. It can be converted from linoleic acid. Arachidonic acid is found in animal fat. It prevents dermatitis but does not promote growth.
>
> *Linolenic acid* is an 18-carbon fatty acid with three double bonds that cannot be synthesized by humans. It does not prevent dermatitis but does promote growth. alpha-Linolenic acid is an omega-3 fatty acid. It can be found in seeds, nuts, and vegetable oils.

Fatty acids are precursors for prostaglandins. This is a critical consideration because the hormone-like substances are produced and used within a tissue rather than transported to other tissues. They affect blood pressure by stimulating the contraction of smooth muscle in blood vessels and regulating the transmission of nerve signals.

When it comes to reproduction, the male's nutritional status is often overlooked, even though it is equally as important as the female's. Males actually require more fatty acids than females. For this reason, nutrients such as fat-soluble vitamins A, D and E are often used in the treatment of prostatic problems with low sperm counts.

Females have greater difficulty digesting fats, and they are more susceptible to biliary stasis (failure of the bile to flow from the liver to the duodenum) than males.

For this reason, women with problem pregnancies should never supplement oils at mealtime, because oils coat the food and make it very difficult to emulsify and digest. It is better to supplement oils between meals or in a dry form whenever possible. Low-fat diets are a problem for fat-deficient women who want to become pregnant. The solution—improve dietary habits and better digestion aided by supplemental plant enzymes.

Lipid-Related Substances

Various lipid-related substances, such as phospholipids and cholesterol, are also essential. Phospholipids are water-soluble. They increase the solubility of fats and keep them in an emulsified state, an extremely important point concerning problem pregnancies. Lecithin, a necessary ingredient in cell walls, is the most common phospholipid.

One of the most important supplements that can be recommended to women with problem pregnancies is a good source of wheat germ that is not in oil form and not defatted.

Sterols are lipid-related substances that include cholesterol and vitamin D. Cholesterol plays an important role in the maintenance of the myelin sheath surrounding the nerve fibers. It is also essential for the formation of sex hormones and bile salts, functions that must be supported during pregnancy. The tendency, unfortunately, is to use prescription drugs, such as statins, that have the opposite effect—they lower cholesterol.

Again, when it comes to reproduction, fats rule.

STAGE TWO:
THE FIRST TRIMESTER

The nutritional status of the woman prior to conception must be known in order to determine her nutritional requirements during pregnancy. Objective tests can be routinely performed to determine the specific needs of a mother-to-be. Physicians often use general nutritional guidelines that are based on national averages to make recommendations for pregnant women. How far the expectant mother is from average, reveals how inappropriate those recommendations tend to be.

Health care providers can have a tremendous impact on the health of expectant parents and their children. Begin with the standard nutritional recommendations and modify them to meet the needs of each individual. Remember, it is not only the components of the diet that count, it is what the patient can digest and assimilate that is important.

Calories and Weight Gain

A pregnant woman must increase her consumption of calories, especially protein, but she does not have to eat for two. The diet should be adequate enough to nourish the fetus without extensive modification. On average, caloric intake should be increased by 300 calories per day. Ideally, an average healthy woman should gain 22 to 29 pounds during pregnancy. It is important to pay special attention to protein and fat digestion, an area of weakness in most women.

In the first trimester, the pregnant woman may not gain weight, especially if she is suffering from morning sickness. The woman usually begins to gain weight during the third month with the most weight gained between the fifth and seventh months. Caution should be used to ensure that weekly weight gain does not exceed 2.2 pounds.

Nutritional Requirements

Many of the hormonal and pregnancy problems encountered during the first months may be related to a protein deficiency. Protein requirements increase only slightly during this period, yet protein digestion and assimilation may be the key to many of the problems encountered.

Some nutrition textbooks recommend an increase of 70–100 grams of daily protein intake. This is a large increase for most women, especially those who already have sluggish biliary function accompanied by low levels of stomach acid. Adequate protein digestion depends on the presence of hydrochloric acid that is needed to activate the protein-digesting enzyme pepsin in the stomach. Unless enough stomach acid enters the duodenum, its rate of flow is reduced and bile thickens.

Iron supplementation should be increased from 30 to 38–40 milligrams per day. Vitamin C is usually recommended to aid iron absorption. An adequate amount of stomach acid must be present to ionize the iron in the stomach, which is essential for absorption. Protein is also essential for iron absorption and transportation even after the iron is ionized.

Calcium intake needs to be increased to at least 1,000 mg per day. This is important for calcification of the baby's bones and teeth. This also helps protect the mother from calcium depletion. Vitamin D can be used to enhance the absorption of calcium. If you are not digesting fat well it doesn't matter how much calcium and Vitamin D you take. The unemulsified fat will bind with calcium, making it insoluble and your body cannot use it.

Digestive and Assimilation Problems

A certain amount of nausea or morning sickness is considered normal during the first three months of pregnancy. Morning sickness indicates that the kidneys are stressed and unable to sufficiently cleanse the blood. Plasma proteins are responsible for detoxifying and transporting waste. Therefore, morning sickness can be eliminated with nutritional support to the kidneys and the lymphatic system.

Edema is also a common problem associated with pregnancy. The common piece of advice offered for this problem is to elevate the legs and mildly reduce salt intake. However, with improved protein digestion and assimilation, the problem will be eliminated altogether.

STAGE THREE:
THE SECOND TRIMESTER

Protein requirements increase even more during the second trimester. Extra protein and calcium are needed to meet the rapid growth of the fetus, the enlargement of the uterus, mammary glands, and placenta, and the increase in maternal blood volume. Even though the demand increases, the ability to digest protein will not improve. In fact, most females do not tolerate large increases in dietary protein.

The second trimester becomes challenging when the excitement of becoming pregnant has waned, and the arrival of the baby becomes increasingly anticipated. The only real excitement during this time comes with the baby's first kick.

The Hormonal System

The anterior pituitary gland, which directs the endocrine system, enlarges at least 50 percent during pregnancy. This allows it to increase its production of the hormones that stimulate the adrenal and thyroid glands.

Improved nutritional support of the adrenal glands is crucial during pregnancy. In addition to its many hormonal responsibilities before pregnancy, the adrenals must now produce an androgenic steroid that is carried to the placenta and converted to estrogen and progesterone. It is imperative that this process is in place by the 12th week in order to replace the role of human chorionic gonadotropin. These hormones prevent spontaneous abortion, loosen the ligaments of the sacroiliac pubis, and prepare breast tissue for lactation.

Adrenocortical secretion is moderately increased throughout pregnancy. It helps mobilize the amino acids of the woman's tissue to be used for synthesis of tissues in the fetus. This represents an apparent need for improved protein ingestion, digestion and assimilation.

During pregnancy, aldosterone secretion is increased three-fold. This causes the retention of excessive amounts of sodium and water, which often leads to hypertension. Aldosterone monitors water volume in the extracellular fluids. Because protein also holds water, aldosterone secretion can be reduced significantly with improved digestion, thus preventing the occurrence of hypertension.

Secretions by the Thyroid Gland

The thyroid gland enlarges about 50 percent during pregnancy and increases the secretion of thyroxine by approximately the same amount. The placenta and the pituitary both secrete thyroid-stimulating hormones. As previously mentioned, the thyroid requires iodine (transported by fatty acids) and protein to produce thyroxine. The use of caffeine and white sugar greatly increases the need for additional thyroxine—a need that a mother-to-be can hardly meet.

Secretion by the Parathyroid Glands

The parathyroid glands enlarge during pregnancy, especially if the mother is calcium (protein) deficient. This enlargement causes calcium resorption from the mother's bones. Parathyroid secretion is greatly increased during lactation because the newborn baby requires more calcium than it did as a fetus.

STAGE FOUR:
THE THIRD TRIMESTER

Many things happen during the final 12 weeks of a pregnancy—much of it having to do with the weight of the baby and mother. By the beginning of this trimester most of the critical fetal formation is complete, or at least well advanced. The baby begins to gain weight rapidly. The mother, on the other hand, will have gained most of her weight between the fifth and seventh months.

The ideal weight gain of 22 to 29 pounds during a pregnancy includes the weight of the baby, the placenta, an enlarged uterus, amniotic fluid, increased blood volume, mammary glands and fat laid down in the tissues in preparation for breast-feeding.

It is important that weekly weight gain is not excessive. Sugar cravings play a prominent role here and are, again, related to poor fat digestion and absorption. The women who have digestive issues prior to pregnancy will struggle with weight once they become pregnant because their already stressed system has even greater metabolic needs to meet.

Edema is a common problem in the latter part of the pregnancy that needs to be carefully monitored in order to rule out pregnancy-induced hypertension. This condition is normally kept under control with sufficient protein intake, digestion and absorption.

Frequent urination is another problem during this trimester. The enlarging uterus exerts pressure against the bladder and results in the urge to urinate. It is important that fluid intake is not reduced. However, caffeine and cola drinks should be avoided because they increase urination.

Constipation is common during pregnancy. This may result from hormonal changes or the heavy compression that the uterus exerts on the intestines. However, the common cause for this condition is the consumption of a diet high in refined sugar and white flour. Plant enzyme supplements will improve protein and fat digestion, thereby curbing sugar cravings and making a diet of whole grains, fresh fruits and vegetables more tolerable.

Desserts, caffeine, cola drinks, and alcohol are high in refined sugar and should be avoided.

There are several consequences of ignoring diet, digestion, and assimilation during pregnancy. Severe toxicity, diagnosed medically as toxemia of pregnancy, or eclampsia, is a life-threatening condition that can develop in the second half of pregnancy. It has no known etiology, or origin, although some believe that it is the result of poor nutrition. The early stages, known as preeclampsia, include signs of high blood pressure, protein in the urine, and excessive edema (not always present).

Despite the lack of an exact etiology, it is apparent that eclampsia severely stresses the organs of detoxification—the liver, kidneys and spleen. The stress to this system can result from poor dietary choices and food enzyme deficiencies. The protein-digesting enzymes are critically important in this area. All nutritional planning during pregnancy should revolve around the prevention of preeclampsia symptoms. This requires an understanding of the role that protein, including its digestion and assimilation, plays in the creation and maintenance of life.

STAGE FIVE:
Postpartum Lactation and Depression

The long-awaited day has arrived. The healthy baby is delivered! It is now time to direct attention to the postpartum nutritional requirements for both mother and her baby.

Lactation

The American Academy of Pediatrics has long advocated the use of breast milk as the primary food source for full-term infants. In 1997, this advisory was extended to include premature infants. The American Academy of Pediatrics recommends that mothers breast-feed their babies for at least one year. The World Health Organization recommends breastfeeding up to age two or beyond.

Many experts believe that breast milk contains a number of compounds that "jump-start" an infant's immune system and help fight off infections. It is interesting to note that many of the immune-enhancing agents that are normally contained in breast milk are found in higher concentrations in mothers who deliver prematurely.

A study published in the peer-reviewed journal *Pediatrics* shows that breast-feeding significantly reduces the occurrence of common infant illnesses such as respiratory tract infections, pneumonia, ear infections, and gastrointestinal tract disorders. In this two-year study of 977 babies, the number of babies that developed pneumonia in the first year of life declined by 33 percent and the cases of gastroenteritis decreased by 15 percent.

It has also been found that preterm infants who are fed breast milk develop significantly fewer infections. In a study of 212 preterm infants with very low birth weights (under three pounds), it was determined that after adjusting for all other factors, the odds for the infants who were fed breast milk to develop an infection had decreased by 57 percent.

If the new mother cannot lactate or produce a sufficient quantity of breast milk, the nutritional cause is invariably a fatty acid deficiency. This deficiency may also manifest in soreness and cracking of the nipple region. An old, yet successful remedy is to massage the area with cocoa butter.

Vitamin deficiencies, such as those of the fat-soluble vitamins A, B, D, and K, can cause health problems.

Research has shown that vitamin A can reduce a child's risk of death from measles. Research has also shown that vitamin A can help treat severe diarrhea in children.

B-vitamins pass from the mother to the baby via breast milk. Deficiencies are more common in vegetarian mothers. In these cases, supplementation is necessary for mother and child.

Vitamin D deficiency is most common when the mother is a vegetarian or lacks adequate sun exposure. Mothers who breast-feed should spend at least 15 minutes in the sunlight daily to increase their vitamin D levels.

Vitamin K deficiency may occur in infants and neonates, including those with malabsorption disorders. This may lead to unexpected hemorrhagic disease. Newborns are often given intramuscular vitamin K shots to prevent this condition.

The American Academy of Pediatrics reported that an iron deficiency may be the result of feeding cow's milk to infants under the age of one. This deficiency can lead to ear infections. Most baby formulas contain iron to prevent such a problem.

Iron and protein deficiencies are often related.

Zinc deficiencies are common in premature infants and children with malabsorption syndromes. Deficiencies are not generally found in breast-fed infants with non-deficient mothers. However, it is believed that the entire human race is borderline zinc deficient. The signs of a zinc deficiency are diarrhea, growth failure, alopecia, irritability, and anorexia. Zinc deficiency is also implicated in skin lesions such as diaper rash and candida manifestations. These implications also indicate a fatty acid deficiency and excessive sugar intake. Individuals who do not digest lipids are those who consume excessive sugars.

Depression

Postpartum depression is a condition that describes a range of physical and emotional changes that many mothers encounter after having a baby. The appearance of any symptom signals exhaustion of the body's ability to maintain homeostasis. This means that normal functions are no longer occurring appropriately. The functions are now occurring too fast, too slow, or incompletely because they are forced to compensate for stress.

Symptoms related to autonomic nervous system imbalance can be understood on the basis of whether the cell is becoming deficient in potassium and hydroxide (alkaline), or calcium and hydrogen (acid). For example, a deficiency of calcium and hydrogen inside the cell produces symptoms of parasympathetic dominance and can be related nutritionally to the inability to adequately digest and assimilate protein and fats. However, a deficiency of potassium and hydroxide inside the cell produces symptoms of sympathetic dominance and can be related nutritionally to excessive ingestion of refined white sugar and white flour products.

The nutritional component of postpartum depression is serotonin deficiency. This deficiency produces symptoms of increased feelings of stress and tension, an exaggerated reaction when startled, a decreased ability to concentrate, and loss of appetite. These symptoms are also consistent with sympathetic dominance. The common nutritional component in both clinical syndromes is exhaustion of intracellular alkaline minerals, primarily potassium. Both conditions are nutritionally related to the inability to properly digest and assimilate fatty acids, with compensation coming in the form of excessive ingestion of foods that are high in sugar and white flour.

Nutritional Etiology

The body produces three neurotransmitters directly from the food we consume. Two amino acids, tyrosine and tryptophan, are used to produce the neurotransmitters that control mood. Dopamine and norepinephrine are alertness chemicals that use tyrosine as a precursor. Serotonin, a calming chemical, uses tryptophan as a precursor.

Almost all protein foods contain much larger amounts of tyrosine than tryptophan. There are a limited number of receptor sites for these amino acids. Due to the abundance of tyrosine, these amino acids are not consumed in equal proportions. Eating protein provides plenty of tyrosine for alertness chemical production; however, an insufficient amount of tryptophan is provided for calming chemical production. Fortunately, after a protein meal, any unused tryptophan is attached to albumin and continues to be carried in the blood. Then, when a high carbohydrate meal is eaten, insulin is released and allows tryptophan to attach to the receptor sites. This increases serotonin production, which exerts a calming effect.

A Continual Reflex Arc

Patients who have difficulty digesting lipids suffer from hydrochloric acid deficiencies and biliary stasis. Invariably they consume excessive amounts of refined simple sugars and function quite well in this state until the symptoms of alkaline mineral deficiency, sympathetic dominance, and serotonin deficiency become evident.

Digestion begins in the mouth with the chewing of food and the addition of saliva that contains water, enzymes, and the alkaline minerals—sodium and potassium. However these salivary secretions are reduced during periods of emotional stress and its resulting conditions, such as fear and anger.

The body is locked into a continual reflex arc and its nutritional components must be addressed. Overall, the key to a healthy pregnancy is improved protein and fat digestion accompanied by a reduced consumption of white sugar and white flour.

> Pregnancy is not just limited to the three trimesters, as commonly believed. Nutritional preparation for creating a life must begin well before conception and continues on after the birth of the child.
>
> An understanding of the five nutritional stages just described can alleviate much of the emotional and physical stress that is associated with pregnancy.

CHAPTER 5

And So It Begins

The Perimenopausal Years

Someone once suggested to me that the upside of a woman's reproductive life cycle—her journey from menarche through her childbearing years—and the downside of her reproductive life cycle, beginning at perimenopause and ending at menopause, are mirror images of one another.

The metaphor works, in the sense that these two phases of a woman's reproductive life cycle are mirror opposites. The hormonal picture is reversed. On one side, her hormonal potential—her ability to produce reproductive hormones—is on the rise, while on the other side, her potential to do so is on the decline.

It's the same body, with symptomatic ups and downs on both sides, seeking normalcy in the midst of continuous hormonal fluctuations, with the birth control pill and hormone replacement therapy acting as opposing forces on both sides of the equation.

Taking the metaphor one step further, with regard to symptoms, nutrition—or a lack of it—is a common denominator. The same deficiency factors we saw driving the four types of

PMS—protein, carbohydrate, lipids and the use of antacids and proton pump inhibitors to shut down stomach acid—also drive symptoms associated with perimenopause. Protein is the major player here too.

And the key to relieving both PMS and perimenopausal symptoms remains the same—nutritional strategies aimed at restoring normal function.

While the symptoms related to perimenopause are not as diffuse or prolific as those related to premenstrual syndrome, these symptoms can be just as life-disrupting, if not more so, because they are inherently perpetual and unpredictable—they do not come and go with a woman's monthly cycle.

And they can last 10 years before a woman finally reaches menopause. I can still hear the scream of one of my female employees when we were discussing an upcoming seminar on women's health, and she heard that perimenopause can be a 10-year sentence.

So here is our middle-aged Juliet, her childbearing years behind her, about to experience her first hot flash.

At what point can she stop taking the birth control pill?

Should she start hormone replacement therapy? If so, when?

These decisions will be made with the help of her primary care provider, but the determination is somewhat arbitrary. Perhaps more important to her health and overall well-being, what nutritional strategies—tailored to her individual needs—can be implemented to restore and maintain normal function and make her journey through this transitional netherworld a more comfortable one?

The Transition Begins

The word perimenopause, which translates literally to "about" or "around" menopause, is used to describe the transitional years before and after a woman's final period. As a medical convenience, perimenopause is technically defined as the time her menses starts to the time when it becomes irregular, until 12 months after her last menstrual bleed. However, because the hormonal changes involved are gradual, both in onset and in termination, the various perimenopause effects often start before and continue after this neatly defined time slot.

During perimenopause, the ovarian production of estrogen and progesterone becomes more irregular, often with wide and unpredictable fluctuations in levels. During this time, fertility diminishes *but* a woman's fertility is not considered to reach zero until her "official" date of menopause, which is determined retroactively—once 12 months have passed after the last appearance of menstrual blood.

Hence the big question: When should a woman stop taking the Pill?

Signs and effects of the menopause transition can begin to appear as early as age 35, though most women don't become aware of this transition until they reach their mid to late 40s, often many years after the actual beginning of the perimenopausal window. The duration of perimenopause, with noticeable bodily effects, can be as brief as a few years, but it is not unusual for this duration to extend to 10 or more years. The actual duration and severity of perimenopause effects—i.e., symptoms—for any individual woman cannot be predicted in advance. Even during the process itself, the course of an individual woman's perimenopausal journey can be difficult if not impossible to predict.

Such is the nature of this journey.

Good News About Symptoms?

When it comes to symptoms, there is both good and bad news.

The good news, again, is that perimenopausal symptoms are not as diffuse or prolific as the different symptoms associated with PMS. The bad news when it comes to perimenopausal symptoms is that there does not seem to be any rhythm or rhyme or reason to them.

> **Unlike PMS symptoms, they're not tied to the menstrual cycle, or any other cycle. perimenopausal symptoms can fluctuate with hormonal ups and downs from day to day, hour to hour. Quite simply, there's no way to know what is coming or when.**

Many women approaching their perimenopause years are advised by their primary care provider to expect a few hot flashes (aka hot flushes) and night sweats as hormone fluctuations commence. However, what often follows these symptoms, sooner rather than later, are unexplained mood swings, vaginal dryness and loss of libido. And what often comes next without warning are heart palpitations, periods of vertigo (dizziness), and very restless sleep night after night, leading to chronic fatigue.

All this may lead to feelings of losing control, to extended periods of anxiety, overwhelming thoughts of doom and dread, even panic attacks in extreme cases. It's little wonder, if these symptoms continue unabated, that a woman may feel she is "losing her mind," or at least losing control of her life.

One minute you're on a quiet familiar beach; the next minute the waves are breaking over you, one after another.

And all this usually starts with the hallmark hot flash.

A Word or Two about Hot Flashes

The hot flash occurs as the body temperature soars upward, reaching a peak very rapidly. The "hot" sensation is not from the initial temperature rise; rather, it is a reaction to the slowness of the body's return to a more normal temperature range.

In some cases, hot flashes can be so strong that they raise the body temperature multiple degrees in a very short period of time. This extreme temperature differential can cause the sufferer to feel weak, break out in a heavy sweat, and experience a rapid heartbeat. Hot flashes, which typically begin in the face or chest but may spread throughout the body, may last two to 30 minutes. The surface of the skin, particularly facial skin, actually becomes hot to the touch and visibly reddened.

Hot flashes can occur a few times a week or dozens of times each day, with the greatest frequency and most intense flashes occurring in warm environments. <u>Hot flashes occurring at night, when estrogen is lowest</u>, are called "night sweats." Some women only experience hot flashes at night.

Despite the discomfort associated with them, hot flashes are not considered harmful by health care providers. In most cases, they can be treated to ease extreme discomfort, using hormone replacement therapy (HRT) or SSRI antidepressants. SSRIs (selective serotonin reuptake inhibitors) affect the brain's use of the neurotransmitter serotonin, which is believed to play a role in regulating body heat. Over-the-counter plant estrogens and herbal remedies are also used to treat hot flashes.

Many women coming to my office wanted nothing to do with drugs, opting instead to dress in heat-dissipating clothing (natural fibers and loose, lightweight clothing), as well as using fans to reduce excessive heat, and staying in cool or air-conditioned rooms.

What causes hot flashes? It's basically the brain trying to get the body to make more estrogen.

Imagine the body as an airplane flying from Los Angeles to New York. As it approaches New York, it goes into a slowly descending glide path. But instead of having a nice smooth approach to the runway and settling down gently into menopause, it encounters a "thunderstorm," and the hypothalamus is busy trying to figure out what is needed to smooth out the rumbling glide path. When the hypothalamus realizes that the body is not producing enough estrogen, it hits the thyroid button to kick up the metabolism, and the arteries expand to increase blood flow.

It's like a niacin flush. If you take 100 or 250 milligrams of niacin, your blood vessels dilate, your body temperature goes up, and your heart rate increases.

The hot flash is the same mechanism.

CHAPTER 5—And So It Begins: *The Perimenopausal Years*

Luckily, not every woman is destined to experience all the symptoms associated with perimenopause, and those who do will not experience the same intensity or duration, simply because every woman is unique.

Let's take a look at the symptoms that have been associated with perimenopause, after which we'll look at the role nutrition—or a lack of it—plays in their exacerbation and what can be done in the way of nutritional strategies to help relieve these symptoms.

> My purpose in writing this book is to share with my readers the role that nutritional deficiencies can play in the symptoms we are going to be talking about. As a practitioner I was focused on my patients' dietary choices and the relationship of these choices to their repetitive, month-after-month, day-after-day, symptomatic patterns. I encourage readers to share the symptoms they are experiencing with their primary care provider.

Mood Changes

Because each woman is unique, so are her experiences as she goes through the gauntlet of symptoms known as the "Change of Life." Some women experience periodic mood swings and irritability. These symptoms may be caused by sleep disruption resulting from hot flashes.

In addition to hot flashes and night sweats, some women also experience anxiety or feeling ill at ease. Even feelings of dread and apprehension are common and are often accompanied by tears.

Some women have difficulty concentrating. Disorientation and mental confusion have also been associated with perimenopause, as well as disturbing memory lapses and fatigue that may border on exhaustion.

Physical Appearance

A woman experiencing perimenopause may notice her body going through subtle (or not-so-subtle) changes. For example, she may be aware of her fingernails as they become soft and break more easily than in her younger days. Her hair may thin (including her pubic hair or hair on her whole body) or there may be an increase in her facial hair. For some women, weight gain is quite common and sometimes difficult to shed.

Headaches and More

A woman's headaches may increase or decrease, often due to digestive issues and increased muscle tension. I found this to be true among my perimenopausal patients, and these headaches could often be relieved with chiropractic care, dietary changes, and improved digestion. The same was true for many cases of tingling in the arms and legs. Breast tenderness also responded to dietary changes and nutritional supplementation.

On the other hand, stiff, sore or aching joints were a repeated complaint. With declining estrogen levels, a woman starts to lose bone more quickly than it can be replaced, which increases her risk of osteoporosis. In a similar way, a woman's skin may become dry, irritated and itchy. Another example is the appearance of pink on the toothbrush. Bleeding gums are usually related to inadequate protein and vitamin C, as is light-headedness or dizziness, or episodes of loss of balance.

Digestion

Around perimenopause, many women experience an occasional bad taste in their mouth, or a change in breath odor. A burning tongue or burning on the roof of the mouth have even been reported. In general, the belly is vulnerable to complaints. For example, increased gastrointestinal distress, indigestion, flatulence, gas pain, bloating and nausea are all common among perimenopausal women. To make matters worse, unpleasant changes in body odor may occur due to hormonal changes, but they are also commonly related to poor digestion and altered bowel movements.

Autonomic Nervous System

Arguably the most common and inconvenient symptom a woman may experience during perimenopause is trouble sleeping through the night, with or without night sweats. This may be due to hot flashes or night sweats, but these often alternate with feelings of being chilled or exposed to the elements. Sleep becomes unpredictable and leads to fatigue on a daily basis.

The list of symptoms goes on. Sometimes a woman may experience an irregular heartbeat or tinnitus in her ears—usually ringing sounds, like bells, whooshing, or buzzing.

It's also a disturbing fact that loss of tissue tone may contribute to incidents of urinary incontinence, especially upon sneezing or laughing. In my experience, as a chiropractor, this symptom is more often due to structural misalignment of the pelvis and not necessarily to hormonal changes.

Menstrual Irregularity

As ovulation becomes more unpredictable, the length of time between a woman's periods may be longer or shorter, her flow may be light to heavy, and she may even skip some periods. A persistent change of seven days or longer in the length of a woman's menstrual cycle may signal early menopause. A space of 60 days or longer between periods is likely to indicate that a woman is in late perimenopause, approaching menopause. Irregular periods are a hallmark of perimenopause and many times nothing to be concerned about. However, medical attention should be sought if any of the following symptoms occur:

- Bleeding is extremely heavy—i.e., changing tampons or pads every hour or two—for two or more hours.
- Bleeding lasts longer than seven days.
- Bleeding occurs between periods.
- Periods regularly occur less than 21 days apart.

Signs such as these may indicate the presence of an underlying issue requiring diagnosis and treatment.

Vaginal Dryness and Loss of Libido

When estrogen levels diminish, vaginal tissues may lose lubrication and elasticity, making intercourse painful. During perimenopause, sexual arousal and desire may change. But for most women who have had satisfactory sexual intimacy before menopause, this will likely continue through perimenopause and beyond.

Decreasing Fertility

As ovulation becomes irregular, a woman's ability to conceive decreases. However as long as she is having periods, pregnancy is still possible. To avoid pregnancy, birth control must therefore be continued until periods have completely stopped for 12 months.

Changing Cholesterol Levels

Declining estrogen levels may lead to unfavorable changes in blood cholesterol levels, including an increase in low-density lipoprotein (LDL)—the bad cholesterol—which contributes to an increased risk of heart disease. At the same time, high-density lipoprotein (HDL)—the "good" cholesterol—decreases in many women as they age, which also increases the risk-of heart disease.

About Early Menopause

While menopause is a normal phase in a woman's life, its' onset is unpredictable and research suggests it may occur earlier than expected when certain risk factors come into play.

Studies have demonstrated that the onset of menopause occurs one to two years earlier in women who smoke, compared with women who don't smoke.

Also, women with a family history of early menopause may experience early menopause themselves.

Treatment for cancer with chemotherapy or pelvic radiation therapy has also been linked to early menopause.

A hysterectomy that removes the uterus but not the ovaries doesn't cause menopause. Even though a woman no longer has periods, her ovaries will still produce estrogen. However, such a surgery may cause menopause to occur earlier than average. Also, it has been found that when one ovary is removed, the remaining ovary may stop working sooner than expected.

A Guessing Game

The big guessing game in perimenopause—when a woman's reproductive self begins its years-long process of winding down estrogen production—is when to stop taking the birth control pill, which is high-dose estrogen, and when to start hormonal replacement therapy, which is low-dose estrogen.

Juliet's doctor would probably like to reduce her estrogen, but as long as she's having periods, there's the risk of an unwanted pregnancy. Doing so also creates problems because you're interfering with normal function. The price one pays in doing so, in terms of symptoms, is dependent on the genetics of each individual woman.

Monitoring body follicle-stimulating hormone (FSH) helps a doctor determine when a woman is about to ovulate, but there's still a lot of guesswork involved, and there's a price to be paid for interfering with normal function.

> **For every action, there's a reaction. It's all about maintaining homeostasis. And in the biochemical world, if you rob Patty, there's a better than even chance you're going to wind up paying Pauline, in terms of side effects.**

At some point, her doctor may want to take Juliet off high-estrogen birth control pills and perhaps put her on low-estrogen hormone replacement therapy to help with her symptoms.

But when?

The benefits and guidelines for estrogen replacement therapy have been well-established for postmenopausal women. However, few guidelines exist for estrogen supplementation during the 10 years of perimenopause.

It's a real balancing act. And there's much to consider.

Besides preventing pregnancy, there are other benefits associated with taking today's low-dose birth control pills.

When the Pill first came out, in the 1960s, it contained 150 micrograms of estrogen. Side effects, such as headaches, nausea and breast tenderness, were far more common back then than they are with today's low-dose birth control pills, which contain 35 micrograms or less of estrogen.

That said, it has been reported that the use of low-dose oral contraceptive pills in women over age 35 provides protection against unwanted pregnancy and maintains a stable hormonal environment while decreasing abnormal menstrual bleeding.

Some of the other health benefits of oral contraceptives include a reduction in bone loss and protection against iron deficiency anemia, dysmenorrhea, benign breast disease, endometrial cancer and epithelial ovarian cancer.

As for cardiac health, low-dose contraceptives probably do not adversely affect blood lipid levels in most women. In one study, total serum cholesterol levels decreased, while high-density lipoprotein (HDL)—the good cholesterol—levels increased. And triglyceride levels, which often rise with high-estrogen oral contraceptives, were not affected in this low-dose estrogen contraceptive study.

Ovarian cancer was a significant concern among the perimenopausal and post-menopausal women who I saw during my practice years in the 1980s and 1990s, even though the actual incidence of ovarian cancer is very low. Unfortunately, at that time, there was no proven screening test, and periodic pelvic ultrasound examinations were not especially helpful.

Studies, however, have indicated that the risk of developing ovarian cancer is reduced in women who have used oral contraceptives compared with women who have never used them. One very large investigation, the Cancer and Steroid Hormone (CASH) study, showed an average 40-percent decrease in the development of ovarian cancer among women who had taken oral contraceptives. A protective effect was observed with as little as three to six months of oral contraceptive use. Use for seven years or longer conferred a 60 – 80 percent reduction in the risk of developing ovarian cancer.

Another benefit of low-dose oral contraceptive use during the perimenopausal years is a reduction in the risk of endometrial cancer. The CASH study reported that after 12 – 23 months of oral contraceptive use, the age-adjusted risk of developing endometrial cancer was 40 percent less than the risk in women who have never used oral contraceptives. After 10 or more years of oral contraceptive use, the risk was found to be 60 percent less.

Low-dose oral contraceptive use also appears to be associated with a significant increase in bone density and a reduction in the risk of a woman developing osteoporosis. Several studies suggest that perimenopausal administration of low-dose oral contraceptive pills can help prevent the acceleration of bone loss and substantially reverse the decrease in bone density and resultant osteoporosis that occurs during the menopausal years.

As we will see, it is possible to improve bone health dramatically with supplemental plant enzymes and dietary changes.

Other suggested benefits of oral contraceptives include protection against benign breast disease, ectopic pregnancy, dysmenorrhea and iron deficiency anemia. Iron deficiency anemia is directly related to protein metabolism, and non-pathological dysmenorrhea also responds well to plant enzyme supplementation and dietary changes, as I will discuss in the last chapter.

Although it was known that oral contraceptive use increased the risk of blood clots during the 1980s and 1990s, no substantial risk of stroke or blood clots was found with the use of low-dose oral contraceptives in healthy young women. In fact, no increased risk of stroke was reported in healthy nonsmoking women, regardless of age.

Today, effective screening for smoking and untreated high blood pressure in perimenopausal women can limit, if not eliminate the risk of arterial diseases associated with the use of low-dose oral contraceptives.

> **So what's the problem with oral contraceptives? Again, it's all about interfering with normal function. That's what the birth control pill is designed to do, in order to insure that a woman does not become pregnant. Since each woman is genetically different, it's a guessing game as to which pill is going to work best for her in terms of side effects.**

Lest we forget, there are alternatives to the birth control pill that prevent pregnancy without interfering with normal hormonal balance. There is one hormone free intrauterine device (IUD) available and there are barrier methods like the diaphragm or cervical cap currently on the market. Long acting reversible contraceptives (LARCs), like IUDs, are being increasingly used, according to a 2015 report by the National Center for Health Statistics. The Dalkon Shield scandal of the 1970s cut way back on IUD use, when 200,000 women were injured, many rendered infertile, and 20 dying from infections. The new numbers show that between 2011 and 2013, 11.6 percent of women were choosing primarily IUDs and to a lesser degree implants to avoid pregnancy.

CHAPTER 5—And So It Begins: *The Perimenopausal Years*

Still, the birth control pill remains the contraceptive of choice, followed closely by female sterilization.

If only the Pill didn't work by interfering with a woman's body seeking its natural hormonal balance, especially during the perimenopausal years, when estrogen is on a wild roller coaster—up some months and down others.

The problem is, medicine and pharmacology are practiced on a curve. It's similar to the way students are graded in college, where some get an A and a B, some get a D, but most are C students. So who is the woman sitting in front of the physician who is in need of birth control or hormone replacement therapy? Where do her individual genetics place her on the treatment curve?

It's an impossible question to answer.

Despite all that pharmacology has to offer, women continue to suffer from inconvenient, if not debilitating symptoms—chronic fatigue being one of the most common—throughout their perimenopausal years.

This is why doctors monitor FSH and serum estradiol (estrogen) levels—to follow a woman's ovulation and predict the onset of menopause, and an appropriate time to stop the Pill and perhaps begin hormone replacement therapy.

Until then, it's a guessing game, as her body seeks its own balance. Remember, some months estrogen is up, other months it's down. So our Juliet could still get pregnant. And, all the medications that pharmacology has to offer to help relieve her symptoms, have side effects!

Which brings us to nutrition.

Visceral or Somatic?

It was the visceral aspect of my chiropractic training at Logan College that led me to nutrition as a possible means of restoring normal function and relieving my patients' symptoms.

Visceral, as described earlier in this book, refers to the physiology of the body—i.e., the way its organs function, including the brain—as opposed to somatic, which taken literally refers to the anatomy, or structure of the body, including the spine.

All the tissues and the organs are connected to each other during embryonic development by the nervous system and the brain. When any organ in this integrated system is stressed for any reason, it sends a signal to the brain, which receives the message and sends back its instructions to the appropriate organ or organ system to compensate, thus maintaining normal function, and homeostasis, as long as it can.

Indeed, as my Grandmother used to say, "Robbing Peter to pay Paul won't work forever." That goes for Patty and Pauline too.

Recalling a critical point, the signal coming back from the brain to the struggling organ goes out on a party line to other areas of the body as well. And so the struggling gall bladder can trigger involuntary muscle contractions around the shoulder. The same interrelationships exist for all tissues of the body, including the reproductive organs.

The relationship between shoulder pain and gallbladder distress is quite common. Unfortunately, it is possible for a vicious cycle of nerve transmission to occur, whereby increased signals from the painful shoulder muscles may be sent back to the biliary system, resulting in reduced blood flow and inability to maintain normal digestive function.

These increased involuntary muscle contractions, both in the shoulder or the chest, and in the abdomen below the liver, can be palpated. It is then only necessary for the skilled practitioner to determine whether the cause is structural, in the shoulder or ribcage, or visceral, due to a digestive difficulty.

Once the cause is known, the treatment becomes obvious.

When the cause is visceral, the involuntary muscle contractions will pass when the digestive problem is resolved. But the muscle contractions will invariably return the next time the patient indulges and stresses her digestive organs.

The effective clinician will have committed to memory the somatic regions (body and spine) that are likely to be affected by nerve transmission signals resulting from visceral dysfunction.

> This is how the science of chiropractic can be used to diagnose hormonal imbalance and restore normal function using nutrition. In other words, you record the outward manifestations of the body's needs—what organ is crying for help—and use nutrition to restore normal function, with the key element being the pre-digestive enzymes needed to deliver that nutrition—protease, amylase, lipase—to the struggling organ system.

And that is how a small-town chiropractor practicing in a rural community came to see so many women with non-pathological menstrual problems. And how he was able to understand whether the *cause* of their symptoms was visceral or structural.

In the end, it's all about giving the struggling organ system what it needs to do its part in maintaining homeostasis. Then, the body will heal itself.

Attention, Intention, and Nutrition

Many of the women who came to my office were seeking so-called alternative therapies because pharmaceutical medicine had not been helpful in relieving their symptoms. They were not seeking manipulative therapy, but rather guidance with dietary changes and nutritional supplementation.

After a careful case history—which included the patient's menstrual history as well as her use of oral contraceptives or hormonal replacement and whether she had been through a partial or complete hysterectomy—I turned my attention to her nutritional status.

I always started by inquiring whether a woman was using antacids, or a prescription medication to reduce or prevent the formation of stomach acid. These cases may require restoration of a normal mucosal lining in the stomach or the small intestine that had become damaged by stress, whether emotional, nutrition, or structural. However, as discussed in the next chapter, reducing or shutting down the production of stomach acid also impairs both protein and fat digestion.

Next, I attempted to identify a causal nutritional deficiency based on the primary nutrients of carbohydrate, protein and lipids.

Armed with my knowledge of the viscero-somatic relationships in the body—the relationships between anatomy, neurology and physiology—I was often able to understand via the patient's symptoms and involuntary muscle contractions why and where her body was crying out for help, and what organ system was under stress.

With this knowledge I was able to help nourish the body in a way that was complementary to the pharmaceutical approach and not competitive with it, delivering specific plant enzymes insuring digestion and assimilation of the nutrients being delivered to the woman's body.

> **The key in all of this came to me with the realization that the symptoms related to perimenopause fell into the same four deficiency types as the symptoms related to PMS—protein, carbohydrate, lipid and the use of proton pump inhibitors.**

This fourfold nutritional dynamic remains the same throughout every stage of a woman's life, from menarche to her post-menopausal years.

Her body changes, and therefore the symptoms change.

So if a woman came to my office complaining that she didn't like protein, that it didn't make her feel good and she wasn't going to eat it, I would explain to her that if she could just digest the protein she was eating, she wouldn't be having the symptoms she was having. If she was a Sugar Bear, I could turn off her sugar cravings in 2 weeks by providing her with the protein energy she needed.

Trying to add a little humor to the situation, I might say something like: "I'm not asking you to eat the north end of a southbound mule. I just need you to eat enough protein, and I will digest it for you." In other words, I was offering enough plant enzymes to do that job.

To a lipid-deficient patient, I would explain that she was not digesting the lipids to make the hormones she needed.

That, and the scientific truth: "You're not getting enough of the fat-soluble vitamins because you're not making enough hydrochloric acid to stimulate the flow of bile."

The nutritional imbalance was the same in perimenopause as the nutritional imbalance in PMS. It was just the *symptoms* that differed.

And the supplementary plant enzymes—the key to relieving symptoms—delivered the nutrition to restore balance and normal function.

The more I practiced this visceral/nutritional approach, the more I learned.

> What it all came down to was whether a woman was eating to her genetic strength or her genetic weakness. That's what makes all this so complex. The body's enzymes are made in the genes. The recipe for making enzymes is written in each person's genetic code. So, again I ask, is she eating to her genetic strength or her genetic weakness?
>
> Does she have the enzymes to digest what she's eating? The body must be nourished.

I found that certain symptoms are likely to be associated with a causal nutritional deficiency based on the primary nutrients—i.e., carbohydrate, protein and lipids—and can be treated accordingly with those nutrients, while other symptoms are "general" and require further investigation to determine the specific cause.

General symptoms include stiff/sore joints, headache, heartburn or indigestion, gas pain/bloating, constipation/diarrhea, anxiety/irritability, restlessness and problems sleeping.

Perimenopausal symptoms are more likely to be identified with a specific causal nutritional deficiency and treated accordingly. These symptoms fall into the same types as PMS symptoms, which I'm repeating here for emphasis:

Carbohydrate-related (PMS-C). This includes decreased secretions in the mouth, nose and eyes; water loss—i.e., dry mouth and skin; the inability to concentrate, muscle cramps during exercise, muscle weakness, patient easily startled, and loss of energy and increased fatigue.

Protein-related (PMS-A). This type would include increased secretions in the mouth, nose and eyes; water gain, involving swelling in the hands and the feet; cold hands and feet; muscle cramps at night; and also menstrual cramps, bleeding gums, and the inability to tolerate exercise.

Lipid-related (PMS-H). This type would include dry skin, scaly rashes, body tremors (non-neurological), and a woman's history of the following major problems:

- Inability to control blood pressure
- Inability to conceive
- Inability to induce labor
- Spontaneous abortion

And so a woman's life comes around full circle, with the same nutritional deficiencies that drove the four types of PMS—protein, carbohydrate and lipids—driving her perimenopausal symptoms.

The nutritional approach to reducing the symptoms of PMS and perimenopause remains the same—nutritional strategies aimed at restoring normal function.

In the next chapter, the mirror image will become complete as our Juliet makes her way from her menopausal to her post-menopausal years.

CHAPTER 6

It's Not Over

Menopause and Beyond

They've been called the "Wisdom Years."

For Dr. Christiane Northrup, menopause represents "an exciting developmental stage—one that, when participated in consciously, holds enormous promise for transforming and healing our bodies, minds, and spirits at the deepest level."

And yet, she goes on to say, the "lifting of the hormonal veil—the monthly cycle of reproductive hormones that tends to keep us focused on the needs and feelings of others—can be both liberating and unsettling."

Indeed, like everything in life, menopause is a two-sided coin.

It's an arrival, a point at which a woman looks back and realizes that she no longer has all of the problems that came with the ability to reproduce. The hormonal fluctuations that began with her first period and continued throughout her fertile years, through perimenopause, right up to her last period, are in the past.

Today's woman has far more to look forward to when she reaches menopause. In 1900, Northrup notes, the average life expectancy for a woman was a mere 40 years. For those who lived beyond it, "menopause was experienced as a signpost of an imminent and inevitable physical decline. But today, with a woman's life expectancy at 84 years, it is reasonable to expect that she will not only live 30 to 40 years beyond menopause, but be vibrant, sharp, and influential as well."

> **Looked at through this lens, menopause becomes a major rite of passage in a woman's life, to be viewed as a great gift, a liberation. It presents an opportunity to reevaluate one's purpose in life, and to change in positive ways.**

Women who celebrate menopause see change not as something to dread, but as an opportunity to embrace what the next stage of life will bring, to move on to greater fulfillment.

The wildly unpredictable hormonal fluctuations of the perimenopausal years are in the past. The plane has landed.

But the story is not over, for the same nutritional factors that came into play during her reproductive years, creating symptoms, will follow a woman into her wisdom years.

It's the same story, from cradle to grave. And with knowledge comes understanding.

Welcome to Menopause

Menopause is the cessation of menstruation and the termination of fertility. The two are not the same thing and may in fact occur at different times. The word climacteric, which derives from the Latin word *climacterics* (critical point in life), refers to the transitional phase—a.k.a. perimenopause—during which time ovarian function and hormone production decline, and the body readapts. Neither menopause nor the climacteric phase should be regarded as a health problem, but rather a natural part of the process of human life.

Advancing age brings with it inexorable changes in ovarian and menstrual function. The average length of a woman's monthly cycle gradually shortens from about 28 days at age 20 to a little longer than 26 days at age 40. At this point, the ovaries begin to lose their ability to produce mature eggs, as well as estrogen and progesterone. Thus, there is the sharp drop in fertility for women over the age of 40. The regular intervals between periods that typically define menstruation for most women become interspersed, with increasing numbers of cycles of shorter and longer duration.

Finally, the interval between periods lengthens and menstruation ceases.

These climacteric "change of life" years leading up to menopause are a time of great emotional as well as physical adjustment. In the United States, the majority of women experience menopause between ages 40 and 55, with the average being age 51.

For several years before menopause, the decline in ovarian hormone production brings changes that are expressed as a variety of discomforting signs and symptoms, as discussed in Chapter 5. The key to understanding the etiology of these symptoms is knowing that during the menopause transition, estrogen production is reduced but does not cease, whereas progesterone production, along with ovulation, does cease entirely at menopause.

This leads to an imbalance—with estrogen free to act untempered by the effects of progesterone. Hence, what Dr. John Lee, who published his conclusions about conventional hormone replacement therapy over a decade ago, has called "estrogen dominance." This imbalance also leads to an array of symptoms including hot flashes, sleep disturbances, poor bladder control, dryness of the vagina, mood swings and irritability. Some women also report weight gain, lack of energy, malaise, forgetfulness, cloudy thoughts, anxiety or panic attacks, sore bones, and general aches and pains.

Then comes menopause, and with it the risk for osteoporosis, a disorder characterized by a slow progressive thinning and loss of calcium content of the bones.

Osteoporosis

Although osteoporosis actually begins in the fourth decade of life in both sexes, it is accelerated in women after menopause. With time, the bones become brittle and more susceptible to fractures from seemingly minor injuries. When the disease is advanced, even coughing, sudden movements, or everyday activities may cause a bone to break. Wrist and hip fractures and collapse of the spinal vertebrae are especially common. This can result in a loss of height and increased thoracic kyphosis, or forward curvature of the spine.

Estrogen deficiency plays a role in post-menopausal osteoporosis, by diminishing the intestinal absorption of calcium. In addition, it increases the loss of calcium from the skeleton. Therefore, osteoporosis is considered to be a calcium deficiency.

And yet, calcium supplementation does not correct this condition.

The drugs used to prevent osteoporosis may actually be doing more harm than good. The stated purpose of biphosphonates (Fosamax®, Boniva®, Reclast®, Actonel®) is to slow bone loss while increasing bone mass, which may prevent bone fractures.

Bone Metabolism: How It Works

> There are two aspects to bone metabolism. One aspect involves osteoblasts, which are bone cells that are continually forming new bone; the other involves osteoclasts, which are continually breaking down and removing older bone. The osteoporosis drugs only block osteoclastic activity.

The result? Old bone accumulates and may lead to a condition known as osteonecrosis, whereby bone breaks down faster than the body can make enough strong, new bone, resulting in increased risk of injury—i.e., fracture. Other serious complications of this condition may include jaw pain, swelling, numbness, loose teeth, gum infection, or slow healing after injury or surgery involving the gums.

Among the many side effects of biophosphonates are: pain, diarrhea, vomiting, headaches and hypertension.

Patients are required to stand upright for at least 30 minutes after taking the drug, and are also instructed not to eat or drink anything but plain water during this period because it can cause serious problems in the stomach or esophagus.

Directions accompanying these drugs advise that they are only part of a complete treatment program that may also include dietary changes, exercise, and the taking of calcium and vitamin supplements.

The key words here are *dietary changes*. Because it is not possible to restore normal function or maintain health using drugs. Drugs are designed to interfere with normal function, and are best used in the treatment of disease. Due to their potential side effects, they should not be recommended for preventing osteoporosis.

This is where the nutritional approach comes in—and the use of plant enzymes.

During my years in practice, I was able to identify three dietary factors that contributed to the development of osteoporosis in my patients. These included problems with carbohydrate, protein and/or lipids—the same three factors underlying PMS and perimenopausal symptoms.

First, there's our Sugar Bear.

> Bone is made up of a protein matrix which contains primarily calcium and phosphorus. The processing of sugars requires phosphorus. A person who consumes excessive amounts of simple sugars is going to be constantly depleting phosphorus and at risk for developing osteoporosis.

Furthermore, inadequately digested complex carbohydrates will disturb the calcium-phosphorus ratio in the blood, causing urinary loss of calcium.

If a person is protein deficient because they are not consuming or digesting enough protein, they will not have enough protein to combine with calcium in the blood, and the calcium will be excreted in the urine rather than transported to and deposited in the bone.

Finally, there are the lipids. When a person is not digesting lipids adequately, these fats will combine with calcium to form insoluble soaps, which will then be passed out of the body in the stool.

With all this in mind, it's no wonder that calcium supplements in themselves are not an effective means of preventing osteoporosis. The more effective course is dietary strategies, including the use of plant enzymes to improve digestion and the use of all three major food substrates—carbohydrates, protein and lipids.

So the same dietary factors that we saw underlying many PMS and perimenopausal symptoms also factor into a woman's risk for developing osteoporosis, as well as other menopausal issues.

This insight would become even clearer to me when I was approached at one of my seminars several years ago by a nurse from a local convent.

The Nun Study

I was speaking at a seminar on women's health and nutrition in Louisville, Kentucky, in 2012. I was talking about a time when I was a young boy growing up in a small town in upstate New York, where my father and mother owned a bakery. One day, my mother asked me to deliver two bags of baked goods to the nuns who lived in a home right next to the church. I was told to go to the back porch, because that's where the kitchen was. When I knocked on the door, one of the nuns came and let me into the kitchen. She talked to me for a little while and I was struck by an incredible sense of peace and tranquility. It was overwhelming.

After my talk, one of the attendees, a retired RN, came up to me and said that she was also a nun. Then she kiddingly told me that not everything is peaceful in a convent. We both laughed.

Later at that same seminar, she came up to me again.

"Dr. Loomis," she said, "this is wonderful information you are teaching us here. I would like to take some plant enzymes back to the convent for a couple of the sisters who I believe could really use them."

She was planning to donate her vacation money to pay for the supplements, but I wouldn't have that. I told her to let me know what she needed and I would send them to her.

Not long afterwards, I shared this story with one of the clinicians I work with, who was at that same seminar.

"I know that nun," she said.

She suggested that as long as I was donating the plant enzymes, she could call the sister and ask her to pick 20 nuns who would be willing to participate in a study. She would then go to the nunnery herself, take patient histories of the 20 participants, and do a palpation exam, looking for soreness. Three months later, she would go back and do the same examination with the same nuns after they had been taking the plant enzymes for that three-month period.

So began our study.

There were 200 retired nuns living at that convent. It wasn't an affluent retirement community. They ate at a cafeteria-style steam table buffet—basic American fare— consisting of meat and potatoes with some vegetables, and a salad bowl one would expect to see on a table for a family of five or six.

The meals were the same every Monday, the same every Tuesday, and so on for every day of the week.

All participants were retired, ages 55 to 90, with numerous health issues, including but limited to: arthritis and digestive issues, severe migraine headaches, chronic fatigue, diabetes, and pain resulting from sciatica, previous surgeries and fibromyalgia, as well as injuries resulting from falls.

And they were all taking various prescription and over-the-counter medications.

> The purpose of this study was to evaluate the effect of adding a mild, pre-digestive plant enzyme supplement to the diet of sedentary senior citizens. With the exception of one 55-year-old participant, all the other women in this specific group were between ages 65 and 90. The average age of the 20 participants was 75.

It was the perfect study group. The all shared a common life style, including living on the same property, partaking of the same cafeteria-style meals prepared by professional dietitians. They also had similar exercise opportunities and the same access to medical supervision and treatment.

Our goal was to give each woman a measured amount of nutritional support in addition to the current dietary choices. No attempt was made to adjust each individual's dietary choices, and the same low-dose pre-digestive formula was given at each meal. This consisted of two capsules containing a balanced dose of protease, amylase, lipase and cellulase plant enzymes to assist them in the digestion of what they ate.

In addition, each participant received—at breakfast and lunch—a capsule of a balanced nutritional supplement containing a very small amount of carbohydrate, protein and lipids from vegetable sources. It was a *very* low dose, given just to make sure they were getting a modicum of nutrients.

The formulas were given at each meal by the cafeteria staff.

Also, no attempt was made to treat the symptoms reported by each individual. The results were reported exclusively by the

CHAPTER 6—It's Not Over: *Menopause and Beyond*

nuns themselves at the end of the three-month period, without any suggestions by the examiner, and without any dietary suggestions.

Two separate examinations were performed—one at the beginning of the study, in July of 2013, prior to anyone receiving the plant enzyme supplements, and again, in October of 2013, after the participants had been taking the supplements for three months.

The examinations included a survey form completed by each nun, listing a chief complaint, if any, and briefly describing any limitations this problem caused in her daily activities. Height, weight, blood pressure and pulse pressure were also recorded at the time of examination, which was done one hour before breakfast or lunch. Each nun was examined following the same meal both months and by the same examiner.

Each patient completed a self-assessment by answering five questions, on a scale of 1 to 10, with 1 being the lowest value, and 10 the highest, or best. The questions asked were the following:

1. What is the level of your energy?

2. How soundly do you sleep?

3. What is the level of your mental clarity and your ability to concentrate?

4. Rate your overall sense of well-being.

5. What is your level of freedom from general aches and pain?

The second part of the study involved the examiner palpating 34 different trigger points on each subject, in the same time-window for each individual nun—one hour after the same breakfast or lunch meal at both the beginning of the study and after three months.

The criteria for palpation and recording of the subject's response followed the guidelines set down by the 2nd World Congress of Myofascial Pain and Fibromyalgia.

Each positive tender point had to meet the following criteria:

- Tender points hurt where pressed, but they do not refer pain to some other part of the body.

- The examiner must use enough pressure to whiten the thumbnail.

- The official definition further requires that tender points must be present in all four quadrants of the body—that is, the upper right and left, and lower right and left parts of your body. Therefore, 34 specific areas of palpation were chosen to be examined.

In addition, the examiner (who was the same person for all 20 subjects and was present at both the July and October examinations) incorporated the following procedure for collecting responses from each nun:

 – Each point was palpated in a circular motion 5–7 times to tolerance of the subject.
 – Participants rated their response for each stress point as:
    0 - Feeling of pressure was normal.
    1 - Discomfort only.
    3 - Pain. No "2" responses were allowed.

Now the Results

For the patient self-evaluation, after three months taking the plant enzyme supplements, average scores were as follows:

- Level of energy went from 5.26 to a 6.9, for a 16.4% improvement.
- Level of sound sleep went from 6.36 to 7.2 for an 8.4% improvement.
- Level of mental clarity/ability to concentrate: 7.1 to 7.7, for a 6.0% improvement.
- Overall sense of well-being went from 7.4 to 8.7, for a 13% improvement.
- Level of freedom from general aches and pains went from 5.4 to 6.6—for a 12.2 % improvement.

This was after just three months!

Nuns weren't given access to their self-assessments from their previous responses.

Now the palpation results.

The total number of sensitive points per patient went from 22 in July to 8.6 in October, for a 61 percent reduction.

And the total soreness per patient went from 70.8 to 15.5, for a 55.3 percent reduction in soreness.

Again, after just three months taking a low-dose plant enzyme formula!

I was stunned. We had done nothing to alter their diet, with the exception of a dose of lipids, protein, carbohydrates and fiber in a capsule, just to make sure each nun got a modicum of nutrition.

All we really did was provide the pre-digestive plant enzymes to assist their digestion of what was basically an food enzyme-deficient diet. Everything was cooked. And they hardly ate any salad.

It was overwhelming to me how successful the study was with such little effort on the part of the nuns.

It was the plant enzymes.

Sooner or later, it all comes down to nutrition.

Epilogue

The Final Word

In writing this book, I have revisited my own learning curve.

When I look back at my first 18 years in practice, I see a time when women kept coming to my office with the same problems—the same recurring symptoms—and I wasn't able to do anything for these women.

First, it started with the young woman arriving at menarche; then all the symptoms associated with PMS and with the birth control pill; followed by the hot flashes, which mark the beginning of the perimenopause years; and finally, the emergence of osteoporosis during the "Wisdom Years."

None of the symptoms made any sense. Not in my mind. Why? Because it all had to do with reproduction, and reproduction is a normal process. So, it follows that there should be no problems, no life-disrupting symptoms associated with it. Why don't we have problems growing up with other normal processes in the body? Why is reproduction such an overwhelming issue for women throughout most of their lives?

Even when it's over, when a woman is no longer menstruating, the life-disrupting symptoms that emerged during her reproductive years may continue to plague her for the rest of her life, while other women don't have any of those symptoms, or at least to a far lesser degree.

So what is the problem with what *should* be a normal biological process?

That's the question that used to drive me crazy.

From the time I finished school until 1980, I lived with that unanswerable question, powerless to help my female patients with their "female problems."

The medical doctor could write a prescription for a medication targeting this or that symptom, but these medications did nothing to restore normal function. And they all carried a suitcase full of unpleasant side effects.

Nutrition was the key. I was certain of that.

I knew that the vast majority of the women I saw were protein deficient, as well as HCl deficient, which impaired their ability to digest both protein and lipids. My laboratory tests confirmed this fact and more. I spent years giving them supplements to improve their protein assimilation and their biliary function—the aforementioned Betaine HCl, and Ox bile salts.

And I added pancreatic enzymes to aid in digestion.

But nothing worked.

Then came Dr. Edward Howell with his plant enzymes. Aha! That was the missing link!

And that's when everything changed. I had the means of diagnosing what each patient's specific nutritional deficiency was, and now I had the means of delivering that nutrition.

For my patients, I had the lab tests, and the physical exam.

Epilogue: *The Final Word*

Before any of this, however, I took a case history of each patient.

Before I examined a woman or ran any kind of test, I could tell exactly what her problem was based on her symptoms.

Did she have increased secretions in her mouth, nose and eyes? Did she have cold hands and feet? Water gain and swelling in her hands and feet? Did she have muscle cramps at night? Pink on her toothbrush? Was she unable to tolerate exercise? Was she stressed out? Was she irritable much of the time? Did she suffer from insomnia, and was she worn out and tired all the time?

The above were all signs of protein deficiency, which was often tied to a calcium deficiency.

Did she have decreased secretions in her mouth, nose and eyes? Did she have water loss, dry mouth and skin? Did she have difficulty concentrating? Did she experience muscle cramps and weakness during exercise? Did she startle easily? Did she suffer from loss of energy and fatigue? Was she eating too much sugar?

All of these were signs of carbohydrate deficiency.

Did she have dry skin? Did she suffer from tremors and uncontrollable blood pressure? Was she unable to conceive a child? Was she unable to induce labor? Did she have a history of spontaneous abortion?

This patient was lipid deficient.

The not-so-obvious became obvious.

A woman would be unable to handle stress. She'd be worn out, suffering from insomnia and unable to conceive, and she would be blaming it all on the stress in her life. It was her husband, her job, her kids, the next door neighbor. More often than not, however, it was her diet. She was protein deficient, carbohydrate deficient, or lipid deficient.

Plant enzymes were the key. Using plant enzyme supplements, I could deliver key essential nutrients past an incompetent digestive system and relieve these patients of their symptoms.

The nun study was proof positive of this. With essentially no change in diet, just the pre-digestive action of the plant enzyme supplements they were given at each meal, their health improved. And, the improvement in symptoms and increase in overall health and well-being was stunning.

I have come to feel very passionately about the fact that women do not have to go through life with all these problems ever again.

And so this book.

Glossary

The following is not intended to replace a medical dictionary, but rather to assist the reader in understanding the terms as they are used within the context of this book.

A

Adrenaline: Brand name for epinephrine, a hormone that causes blood vessels to narrow and the blood pressure to increase.

Adrenocorticotropic hormone (ACTH): A hormone that is produced by the anterior lobe of the pituitary gland and that stimulates the secretion of cortisone, aldosterone, and other hormones by the adrenal cortex.

Aldosterone: A steroid hormone secreted by the adrenal cortex that regulates the salt and water balance in the body.

Amenorrhea: Abnormal absence or suppression of menstruation.

Anatomy: The structural makeup especially of a person or animal.

Anemia: A condition in which the blood is deficient in red blood cells, in hemoglobin, or in total volume.

Anxiety: An abnormal and overwhelming sense of apprehension and fear often marked by physiological signs (such as sweating, tension, and increased pulse), of doubt concerning the reality and nature of the threat, and of self-doubt about one's capacity to cope.

Assimilation: The incorporation or conversion of nutrients into protoplasm that in animals follows digestion and absorption, and in higher plants involves both photosynthesis and root absorption.

B

Bile: A clear yellow or orange fluid produced by the liver. It is concentrated and stored in the gallbladder, and is poured into the small intestine via the bile ducts when needed for digestion. Bile helps in alkalinizing the intestinal contents, and it plays a role in the emulsification, absorption, and digestion of fat.

Biliary: Pertaining to the bile, to the bile ducts, or to the gallbladder.

Bisphosphonates: A class of drugs that prevent the loss of bone mass, used to treat osteoporosis and similar diseases.

C

Capillary fragility: A measure of the resistance to rupture of the small blood vessels (capillaries), which would lead to leakage of red blood cells into tissue spaces.

Carbohydrate: A substance found in food that is composed of simple sugars (from fruits, dairy products, grains and flour, white sugar, honey, molasses, and maple syrup to name a few), complex starches (vegetables), and fiber.

Corpus luteum: A yellowish mass of progesterone-secreting endocrine tissue that forms immediately after ovulation from the ruptured follicle in the mammalian ovary.

Climacteric: A major turning point or critical stage.

D

Digestion: The process by which a substance (food) is divided into two or more substances by enzymes. Water is used in the process.

Disease: Illness or sickness that indicates an inability of the body to maintain normal function(s).

Dopamine: A naturally occurring sympathetic nervous system neurotransmitter that is the precursor of norepinephrine.

Drospirenone: A synthetic progestogen that is used in birth control pills in combination with ethinyl estradiol.

Drug: Any substance other than food used for the diagnosis, alleviation, treatment, or cure of disease.

Dysmenorrhea: Painful menstruation.

E

Ectopic Pregnancy: Development of a fertilized egg elsewhere than in the uterus (as in a fallopian tube or the peritoneal cavity).

Edema: An abnormal excess accumulation of serous fluid in connective tissue or in a serous cavity.

Emulsify: To produce an emulsion by dispersing one fluid, in the form of small globules, in another fluid.

Endometrium: The mucous membrane forming the inner layer of the uterine wall.

Enuresis: An involuntary discharge of urine; incontinence of urine.

Enzyme: Organic catalysts that are composed of protein combined with either a mineral, vitamin, or part of a vitamin.

They are responsible for performing chemical changes in the body. As nutritional supplements they can be sourced from plants or animals.

- Plant enzymes have a much wider pH range of activity, roughly 3.0 to 9.0 and are active in the entire G.I. tract.
- Pancreatic (animal) enzymes work in a narrower range of activity, roughly 7.0 to 9.0 and are not active in the stomach.

Enzyme Nutrition: The process of supplementing naturally occurring plant enzymes into the diet to replace those that are removed or deficient in the modern diet.

Epinephrine: A hormone that causes blood vessels to narrow and the blood pressure to increase.

Estradiol: A natural estrogenic hormone secreted chiefly by the ovaries, is the most potent of the naturally occurring estrogens, and is administered in its natural or semisynthetic esterified form especially to treat menopausal symptoms.

Estrogen: Any of various natural steroids (as estradiol) that are formed from androgen precursors, that are secreted chiefly by the ovaries, placenta, adipose tissue, and testes, and that stimulate the development of female secondary sex characteristics and promote the growth and maintenance of the female reproductive system.

Etiology: The cause of a disease or abnormal condition.

Extracellular fluid: The interstitial fluid and the plasma, constituting about 20 percent of the weight of the body.

F

Fallopian tube: Either of the pair of tubes that carry the egg from the ovary to the uterus.

Fatigue: Weariness or exhaustion from labor, exertion, or stress.

Fats or Lipids: A semisolid substance found in food and composed of glycerol (a sweet-tasting oil) and fatty acids (any acid derived from fat).

Follicle: A vesicle in the mammalian ovary that contains a developing egg surrounded by a covering of cells.

Follicle-stimulating hormone (FSH): A hormone from an anterior lobe of the pituitary gland that stimulates the growth of the ovum-containing follicles in the ovary.

Follicular phase: The phase during which the ovarian follicle develops during the menstrual cycle.

Food: Any substance usually eaten by humans for nourishment. Raw food contains protein, carbohydrates, fats or lipids, vitamins, minerals, and enzymes.

G

Gamma globulin: A protein fraction of blood rich in antibodies.

H

Hemoglobin: The part of blood that contains iron, carries oxygen through the body, and gives blood its red color.

Homeostasis: Any self-regulating process by which biological systems tend to maintain stability while adjusting to conditions that are optimal for survival.

Hormone Replacement Therapy (HRT): The administration of estrogen often along with a synthetic progestin especially to ameliorate the symptoms of menopause and reduce the risk of postmenopausal osteoporosis.

Hot flashes or Hot flushes: A sudden brief flushing and sensation of heat caused by dilation of skin capillaries usually associated with menopausal endocrine imbalance.

Human chorionic gonadotropin (hCG): A glycoprotein hormone similar in structure to luteinizing hormone that is secreted by the placenta during early pregnancy to maintain corpus luteum function and is commonly tested for as an indicator of pregnancy.

Hydrochloric acid: A very strong acid formed by the combination of H+ (hydrogen) and Cl- (chloride) ions to form stomach acid.

Hypothalamus: An organ in the brain that is primarily involved with regulating the autonomic nervous system and the hormonal system of the body, the two major control mechanisms by which the body maintains its normal functions. It also influences our sense of taste and smell.

Hypothyroidism: A condition characterized by insufficient thyroid hormone, weight gain, lack of energy, and need for unusual amounts of sleep.

Hysterectomy: Surgical removal of the uterus.

I

Incontinence: Inability of the body to control the evacuative functions.

Inhibin A: A peptide hormone secreted by the follicular cells of the ovary that inhibits secretion of follicle stimulating hormone from the anterior pituitary.

Insulin: A protein pancreatic hormone that is produced by the pancreas and is necessary for the normal use of glucose by the body.

Intervertebral disc: A layer of cartilage separating adjacent vertebrae in the spine.

Intrauterine device (IUD): A device inserted and left in the uterus to prevent pregnancy.

Ionized calcium: The ionized, unbound, noncomplexed fraction of serum calcium that is biologically active.

J

K

L

Lactase: Simple sugar digesting enzyme (disaccharidase) that digests milk sugar (lactose).

Lipase: A fat digesting enzyme.

Lipids or Fats: A semisolid substance found in food and composed of glycerol (a sweet-tasting oil) and fatty acids (any acid derived from fat).

Luteal phase: The portion of the menstrual cycle that begins with the formation of the corpus luteum and ends with the start of the menstrual flow, usually 14 days in length.

Luteinizing hormone (LH): A hormone secreted by the anterior lobe of the pituitary gland that in the female stimulates ovulation and the development of corpora lutea.

M

Maltase: Simple sugar digesting enzyme (disaccharidase) that digests the sugar found in grains (maltose), such as wheat.

Menarche: The beginning of the menstrual function; especially the first menstrual period of an individual.

Menopause: The natural cessation of menstruation occurring usually between the ages of 45 and 55.

Menstruation: A discharging of blood, secretions, and tissue debris from the uterus that recurs in nonpregnant humans and other primate females of breeding age at approximately monthly intervals.

Metabolize: To undergo metabolism, the breaking down of carbohydrates, proteins, and fats into smaller units.

Mineral: Inorganic materials found in the earth's crust. They cannot be made in the human body. They are found in small quantities in food and are essential for human function and health.

Mucilage: A gelatinous substance of various plants (as legumes or seaweeds) that contains protein and polysaccharides and is similar to plant gums.

N

Neurology: A branch of medicine concerned especially with the structure, functions, and diseases of the nervous system.

Niacin: An acid of the vitamin B complex that is found widely in plants and animals.

Night Sweats: Profuse sweating during sleep, often associated with menopause.

Nutrition: The process of ingesting food and converting it into energy or using it to repair body tissue.

O

Oliguria: Reduced excretion of urine.

Oocyte: An immature ovum, or egg cell.

Osteoblast: A bone-forming cell.

Osteoclast: Any of the large multinucleate cells closely associated with areas of bone resorption.

Osteonecrosis: Death of living bone.

Osteoporosis: A condition that affects especially older women and is characterized by decrease in bone mass with decreased density and enlargement of bone spaces producing porosity and brittleness.

Ovulation: The discharge of a mature ovum from the ovary.

P

Palpation: The art of examining the body by using the hands to feel muscle contractions.

Paresthesia: A sensation of pricking, tingling, or creeping on the skin that has no objective cause.

Perimenopause: The period around the onset of menopause that is often marked by various physical signs (as hot flashes and menstrual irregularity).

Pepsinogen: The inactive precursor to pepsin, formed in the chief cells of the mucous membrane of the stomach and converted to pepsin by hydrochloric acid during digestion.

Physiology: A branch of biology that deals with the functions and activities of life or of living matter (as organs, tissues, or cells) and of the physical and chemical phenomena involved.

Pituitary gland: A gland at the base of the brain that produces several hormones of which one affects growth.

Plasma proteins: Any of the various dissolved proteins of blood plasma, including antibodies and blood-clotting proteins that act by holding fluid in blood vessels by osmosis.

Precursor: a substance, cell, or cellular component from which another substance, cell or cellular component is formed especially by natural process

Premenstrual syndrome (PMS): A varying constellation of symptoms manifested by some women prior to menstruation that may include emotional instability, irritability, insomnia, fatigue, anxiety, depression, headache, edema, and abdominal pain.

Progesterone: A female steroid sex hormone that is secreted by the corpus luteum to prepare the endometrium for implantation and later by the placenta during pregnancy to prevent rejection of the developing embryo or fetus.

Protease: Protein digesting enzyme.

Protein: A substance found in food that contains nitrogen and is composed of amino acids. Examples of protein-rich foods include meats, cheese, and eggs.

Q

R

Receptor site: A chemical group or molecule (as a protein) on the cell surface or in the cell interior that has an affinity for a specific chemical group, molecule, or virus.

Reflex arc: The complete nervous path involved in a reflex.

S

Selective Serotonin Reuptake Inhibitor (SSRI): A class of drugs that are typically used as antidepressants in the treatment of major depressive disorder and anxiety disorders.

Serotonin: A naturally occurring derivative of tryptophan found in platelets and in cells of the brain and the intestine. Serotonin is released from platelets on damage to the blood vessel walls. It acts as a potent vasoconstrictor.

Somatic: Of, relating to, or affecting the structure of the body.

Stress: Any mechanical, chemical, or emotional stimulus that exhausts the normal processes of the human body.

Sucrase: Simple sugar digesting enzyme (disaccharidase) that digests the sucrose found in foods such as white sugar, molasses, honey, maple syrup, or white flour.

Symptom: Any sensation experienced by a person that is indicative of a departure from normal function or structure.

Syncope: Loss of consciousness resulting from insufficient blood flow to the brain; faint.

T

Testosterone: Male hormone (released primarily from interstitial cells of testes), but also from adrenal cortex and ovaries, in much smaller amounts.

Thoracic kyphosis: Exaggerated outward curvature of the thoracic region of the spine resulting in a rounded upper back.

Thyroxin: An iodine-containing hormone that is an amino acid produced by the thyroid gland as a product of the cleavage of thyroglobulin, increases metabolic rate, and is used to treat thyroid disorders.

u

Uterus: The organ in women in which babies develop before birth.

V

Vertigo: A sensation of motion which is associated with various disorders (as of the inner ear) and in which the individual or the individual's surroundings seem to whirl dizzily.

Visceral: Of, or relating to, the internal organs.

Vitamin: Organic substances that cannot be made in the human body. They are found in small quantities in food and are essential for normal human function and health.

W

X

Y

Z

Selected Bibliography

Introduction

Loomis, Howard F., Jr. *Enzymes: The Key to Health.* Madison, WI: 21st Century Nutrition Publishing. 1999.

Loomis, Howard F., Jr. *The Enzyme Advantage: For Health Care Providers and People Who Care About Their Health.* Madison, WI: 21st Century Nutrition Publishing. 2015.

Chapter 1

Frank, Robert T. "Hormonal Causes of Premenstrual Tension." New York Academy of Medicine, 1931. Note: The actual term premenstrual syndrome first appeared in an article in the British Medical Journal in 1953.

Romans S. , Clarkson R., Einstein G., Petrovic M., Stewart D., "Mood and the menstrual cycle: a review of prospective data studies," *Gend Med.* 9(5): 361-384. October 2012

Mayo Clinic on PMS: Accessed at http://www.mayoclinic.org/diseases-conditions/premenstrual-syndrome/basics/causes/con-20020003

Johnson, Susan R., M.D., "200 different symptoms associated with PMS" University of Iowa 2012. Accessed at http://primarypsychiatry.com/the-epidemiology-of-premenstrual-syndrome/

Palmer, D.D. *The Chiropractic Adjuster.* Portland Printing House. 1910. Note: D.D. Palmer founded the field of chiropractic in 1895.

Society for Menstrual Cycle Research. On "cycle-stopping" contraception." Annual Meeting June 2007, Vancouver.

Cannon W.B. *Bodily Changes in Pain, Hunger, Fear and Rage.* New York, NY: D. Appleton & Company; 1915.

Cannon W.B. *The Way of an Investigator: A Scientist's Experiences in Medical Research.* New York, NY: W. W. Norton; 1945:130–145.

Cannon W.B. The role of emotions in disease. *Ann Intern Med.* 1936; 9:1453–1465 Note: The word homeostasis was first coined by American physiologist Walter B. Cannon in 1930. Accessed http://www.ncbi.nlm.nih.gov/pmc/articles/PMC1447286

Selye, Hans, M.D., *The Stress of Life*. New York, McGraw-Hill Book Company, Inc. 1956.

Davis, Adelle. *Let's Get Well*. 1965. Accessed at www.adelledavis.org

Howell, Edward, *Enzyme Nutrition: The Food Enzyme Concept*. Avery Publishing Group, Garden City, NY: p. 1-13. 1985.

Howell, Edward. *Food Enzymes for Health and Longevity*, Second Edition, Twin Lakes, WI: Lotus Press, p. 8. March 1994.

Sandburg, Carl. *Life of Lincoln: The Prairie Years and The War Years*. Brilliance Audio (MP3 version) June 3, 2014.

Allison, Anthony. "Lysosomes and Disease." *Scientific American*, November 1967.

Chapter 2

Witcombe, Christopher L.C. "Eve and the Identity of Women." Accessed: http://witcombe.sbc.edu/eve-women

Davis, Elizabeth, "The Menarche Rite," *Blood Mysteries*. Accessed at http://elizabethdavis.com/articles/blood-mysteries

Christiane Northrup, M.D. *Women's Bodies, Women's Wisdom*. Bantam. 4th Edition. June 2010, Accessed at www.drnorthrup.com

Waterson, David. "Sir James MacKenzie." Br Med J. 1925 March 7; 1(3349): 482. Accessed at http://www.ncbi.nlm.nih.gov/pmc/articles/PMC2226510

Selye, Hans. *The Stress of Life*. New York, McGraw-Hill Book Company, Inc. 1956.

Chapter 3

Our Bodies, Ourselves. "Brief History of Birth Control." Accessed at http://www.ourbodiesourselves.org/health-info/a-brief-history-of-birth-control

Medical News Today. "10 Most Common Birth Control Pill Side Effects." Accessed at http://www.medicalnewstoday.com/articles/290196.php

Deshpande S, Basil MD, Basil DZ. "Factors influencing healthy eating habits among college students: an application of the health belief model." Health

Mark Q. Apr-Jun; 26 (2) 2009. Accessed at http://www.ncbi.nlm.nih.gov/pubmed/19408181

Abraham, G. E. Nutritional factors in the etiology of the premenstrual tension syndromes. *The Journal of Reproductive Medicine*, 28, 446–464. 1983.

Thys-Jacobs, S. "Micronutrients and the premenstrual syndrome: the case for calcium." *J Am Coll Nutr* Apr: 19(2):220-227. 2000 Accessed at http://www.ncbi.nlm.nih.gov/pubmed/10763903

Chapter 4

Centers for Disease Control and Prevention, National Center for Health Statistics. "On Infertility." Accessed at http://www.cdc.gov/nchs/fastats/infertility.htmInfertility statistics

U.S. Department of Health and Human Services (HHS). *The Surgeon General's Report on Health and Nutrition*. Washington, DC. HHS Public Health Service. HHS Publication No. 88-50210. 1988

Wright, Bauer, et al. *Pediatrics*. 1998. Note: It has also been found that preterm infants who are fed breast milk develop significantly fewer infections.

Chapter 5

Romans S. , Clarkson R., Einstein G., Petrovic M., Stewart D., "Mood and the menstrual cycle: a review of prospective data studies," *Gend Med*. 9(5):361-384. October 2012

Mayo Clinic on PMS: Accessed at http://www.mayoclinic.org/diseases-conditions/premenstrual-syndrome/basics/causes/con-20020003

Chapter 6

Lee, John D. "estrogen dominance." Accessed at http://www.johnleemd.com/saliva-hormone-testing.html

INDEX

A
acid-alkaline balance (pH) 22
acne 14, 70, 81
acupuncture 2, 95
adrenaline 77
adrenocorticotropic hormone (ACTH) 86, 163
alcohol 72, 103, 104, 114
aldosterone 86, 112, 163
amenorrhea 50, 51, 66
amino acids 52, 53, 55, 78, 112, 118, 119, 173
amylase 31, 33, 96, 139, 154
anatomy 17, 138, 141
anemia 50, 51, 75, 100, 134, 135
antibodies 59, 77, 167, 172
antidepressant 41
anxiety 2, 13, 14, 79, 80, 81, 98, 125, 127, 143, 148, 172, 173
arthritis 31, 153
assimilation 29, 30, 104, 105, 109, 111, 112, 114, 115, 141, 160
asthma 14
autonomic 23, 25, 53, 118, 168

B
backache 14
Beta Jewish women 45
bile 29, 82, 87, 99, 100, 101, 107, 108, 110, 142, 160, 164
biliary 87, 88, 96, 101, 107, 109, 119, 139, 160
biochemical 53, 133
biphosphonates 149
bleeding 12, 13, 38, 47, 49, 51, 57, 60, 71, 133, 144
bloating 1, 14, 40, 61, 86, 129, 143
blood tests 25, 27, 33, 39, 78, 81
Bone Metabolism 149
brain 18, 20, 23, 24, 25, 53, 55, 103, 126, 138, 168, 172, 173, 174
breasts 46, 58, 70

C
calcium 2, 22, 24, 27, 34, 37, 39, 40, 41, 54, 60, 62, 78, 79, 80, 81, 82, 87, 89, 98, 99, 100, 110, 111, 113, 118, 148, 149, 150, 151, 161, 169, 179
Cannon, Walter B. 21, 177
capillary fragility 14, 164
carbohydrate 14, 15, 30, 52, 53, 59, 83, 86, 91, 119, 122, 141, 143, 144, 150, 154, 161, 162, 164
carbohydrate deficiency 161
caregiver 54
case history 79, 140, 161

cells 21, 22, 23, 26, 27, 36, 37, 52, 53, 54, 55, 59, 62, 68, 99, 149, 163, 164, 167, 169, 171, 172, 173, 174

cellular metabolism 54

cellulase 31, 33, 96, 154

central nervous system 12, 14, 15, 48, 79, 87

Change of Life 127

chiropractor 9, 17, 19, 20, 28, 36, 130, 140

cholesterol 22, 107, 108, 131, 134

chronic 20, 31, 32, 34, 36, 51, 54, 55, 56, 65, 86, 94, 125, 137, 153

circulatory system 18

climacteric 146, 147

common denominator 33, 121

constipation 14, 70, 85, 143

contraceptives 50, 69, 71, 134, 135, 136, 140

contractions 18, 20, 25, 27, 36, 39, 40, 51, 54, 81, 84, 138, 139, 141, 171

corpus luteum 67, 68, 168, 170, 173

cortisone 163

cramps 1, 2, 3, 14, 38, 40, 60, 78, 80, 99, 143, 144, 161

cycle 1, 12, 13, 15, 16, 17, 38, 43, 45, 47, 48, 49, 50, 51, 61, 64, 65, 66, 67, 69, 71, 74, 75, 88, 92, 102, 121, 122, 124, 130, 138, 145, 147, 167, 170, 177, 179

D

degreasing 99

depression 3, 11, 13, 15, 70, 71, 87, 88, 90, 100, 103, 117, 118, 172

dermatomes 19, 20

diabetes 31, 51, 153

diarrhea 116, 117, 143, 150

diet 3, 31, 32, 39, 56, 60, 61, 70, 72, 75, 76, 79, 82, 85, 86, 99, 103, 104, 106, 109, 114, 154, 157, 158, 162, 166

dietary changes 6, 95, 96, 102, 128, 135, 140, 150

digestion 6, 15, 23, 29, 31, 32, 33, 34, 75, 76, 80, 85, 86, 87, 88, 89, 91, 96, 100, 101, 102, 104, 105, 107, 109, 110, 111, 112, 113, 114, 115, 120, 128, 129, 140, 141, 151, 154, 158, 160, 164, 172

disease 6, 12, 14, 17, 24, 25, 26, 31, 35, 36, 51, 74, 76, 97, 117, 131, 134, 135, 148, 150, 165, 166, 177

domino effect 101

dopamine 59, 119, 165

drospirenone 70, 71, 165

drug 17, 30, 36, 63, 150

duodenum 107, 110

Dyak women 44

Dysmenorrhea 51, 165

E

ectoderm 18
ectopic pregnancy 135
edema 14, 40, 78, 86, 114, 172
Egyptians, ancient 45
embryonic layers 18
emotional roller coaster 12, 46, 60, 85
emulsify 82, 107
endocrine system 23, 111
endoderm 18
endometrium 67, 76, 173
energy 1, 4, 15, 22, 23, 25, 33, 48, 49, 52, 53, 54, 55, 58, 59, 65, 83, 100, 101, 142, 143, 148, 155, 157, 161, 168, 171
energy bank account 55
enuresis 14
enzyme 6, 31, 32, 33, 70, 75, 81, 85, 86, 96, 110, 114, 115, 135, 154, 155, 157, 158, 162, 169, 170, 173, 174, 189
- plant enzymes 6, 2, 3, 4, 6, 33, 36, 37, 38, 60, 62, 82, 87, 89, 102, 107, 135, 141, 142, 150, 151, 152, 153, 154, 158, 160, 166
enzyme-deficient diet 158
Enzyme Nutrition 31, 166, 178
epinephrine 59, 163
estradiol 48, 137, 165, 166
estrogen 12, 13, 14, 16, 46, 48, 49, 65, 67, 68, 69, 77, 79, 80, 81, 92, 111, 123, 125, 126, 128, 130, 131, 132, 133, 134, 137, 147, 148, 168, 179

etiology 114, 147, 179
Eve 43, 45, 48, 62, 178
exercise 50, 59, 60, 64, 143, 144, 150, 154, 161
extracellular fluid 22, 24
eye complaints 14

F

fallopian tube 67, 69, 93, 165, 167
fatigue 13, 20, 75, 125, 128, 129, 137, 143, 153, 161, 172
fats 3, 29, 31, 53, 58, 59, 82, 89, 99, 101, 107, 108, 118, 151, 167, 170
fatty acids 87, 106, 107, 112, 118, 167, 169
fertility pills 106
fertilization 95, 106
fiber 157, 164
follicle-stimulating hormone (FSH) 66, 67, 101, 132, 137, 167
follicular phase 66
food 22, 28, 30, 31, 32, 33, 34, 72, 73, 96, 107, 115, 118, 119, 151, 158, 164, 165, 167, 169, 170, 171, 173, 175, 189
- cooked and processed 31
Food Enzyme Concept 31, 178
forbidden fruit 43
Frank, Robert T. 12, 177
fruits 114, 164

G
gall bladder 18, 138
gamma globulin 59
gas 129, 143
gastrointestinal tract 116
genetics 58, 65, 132, 137
glucose 52, 53, 55, 59, 65, 169
glycogen 52, 55
Goldin, Claudia 68
Greece 45

H
headache 40, 143, 172
Head, Henry 19, 20
health care providers
  72, 78, 103, 126
heartburn 88, 143
heart rate 23, 126
hemoglobin 59, 99, 100, 163
herbs 30, 89, 95
homeostasis 21, 23, 24, 26, 27,
  52, 53, 54, 78, 101, 117,
  133, 138, 140, 177
hormonal imbalance 50, 139
hormone replacement therapy
  (HRT) 126, 168
hot flash 122, 124, 125, 126
Howell, Edward 31, 32, 33, 60,
  62, 160, 178, 189
Human chorionic gonadotropin
  (hCG) 68, 112, 168
hydrochloric acid 32, 82, 100,
  101, 110, 119, 142, 172
hypothalamus 23, 53, 66, 126
hypothyroidism 86, 168
hysterectomy 132, 140

I
incontinence 129, 165
indigestion 129, 143
infertility 93, 94, 97, 98, 179
inflammation 27, 36, 37
inhibin A 67, 169
insulin 59, 77, 83, 119, 169
intervertebral discs 29, 169
intestine 32, 34, 140, 164, 173
  - small intestine
    32, 34, 140, 164
  - large intestine 31
intracellular fluid 22
intrauterine device (IUD)
  51, 136, 169
in vitro fertilization 95
involuntary muscle contractions
  18, 20, 25, 27, 39, 54, 81,
  84, 138, 139, 141
ionized calcium 80
iron deficiency
  75, 99, 117, 134, 135

J
Juliet 63, 64, 79, 88, 90, 91, 92,
  122, 132, 133, 137, 144

K
kidneys 83, 84, 86, 110, 115

L
lactase 86, 169
lactation 74, 103, 106, 112, 113
lactose 169
Lillard, Harvey 19
lipase 31, 33, 82, 85, 86, 87, 96,
  139, 154

lipids 30, 52, 53, 56, 59, 65, 117, 119, 122, 141, 142, 143, 144, 150, 151, 154, 157, 160, 167
luteal phase 13, 67, 76, 170
luteinizing hormone (LH) 66, 67, 101, 168, 170
lymphatic system 18, 110

M
MacKenzie, James 19, 20, 178
malnutrition 75, 76
maltase 86
medical condition 12
menarche 43, 44, 45, 46, 48, 57, 62, 64, 80, 92, 121, 141, 159, 170, 178
menopause 121, 122, 123, 126, 130, 131, 132, 137, 145, 146, 147, 148, 168, 171, 172
menstruation 9, 12, 17, 45, 46, 49, 50, 51, 56, 60, 66, 67, 76, 99, 146, 147, 163, 165, 170, 172
menstruation huts 45
metabolic rate 54, 87, 174
metabolize 83, 84
minerals 1, 30, 33, 83, 84, 86, 100, 118, 119, 167
motor reflexes 20
mucilage 89
muscle contractions 18, 20, 25, 27, 36, 39, 40, 54, 81, 84, 138, 139, 141, 171
musculoskeletal system 3, 18

N
neurology 141, 171
neurotransmitters 77, 118, 119
New York, East Aurora 57
niacin 126
night sweats 124, 125, 127, 129
Northrup, Christiane 47, 48, 49, 65, 145, 178, 179
Nun Study 152, 162
nutrition 6, 2, 3, 11, 15, 16, 17, 25, 26, 30, 31, 33, 41, 45, 47, 49, 51, 54, 60, 61, 62, 65, 72, 74, 75, 81, 93, 96, 97, 98, 102, 103, 104, 105, 109, 114, 121, 127, 137, 138, 139, 140, 142, 152, 157, 158, 160, 166, 171, 177, 178, 179
nutritional deficiencies 27, 91, 94, 97, 101, 127, 144

O
oliguria 14
oocyte 67
oral contraceptives 50, 71, 134, 135, 136, 140
organ system 138, 139, 140, 141
osteonecrosis 149
osteoporosis 64, 128, 135, 148, 149, 150, 151, 159, 164, 168
ovulation 13, 46, 47, 48, 49, 51, 59, 67, 69, 88, 93, 99, 130, 131, 137, 148, 164, 170

P
Palmer, D.D. 19, 177
palpation
    13, 25, 124, 153, 156, 157

pancreas 20, 23, 31, 88, 99, 169
pancreatic enzymes 32, 160
parasympathetic 53, 118
paresthesia 14
pastatarians 84
pepsin 32, 82, 89, 110, 172
pepsinogen 82, 89
perimenopause 121, 122, 123, 124, 127, 128, 129, 130, 131, 132, 133, 141, 142, 144, 145, 147, 159
perspiration 23
pH 22, 23, 39, 79, 166
pharmacology 15, 137
phases of the moon 47
physiology 3, 17, 138, 141
pill, the 8, 9, 66, 68, 84, 91, 92, 123, 133, 137
  - birth control pill 16, 66, 68, 70, 86, 90, 92, 97, 121, 122, 132, 133, 136, 137, 159, 165
  - pill 8, 66, 68, 69, 71, 92, 121, 122, 132, 136, 137, 159
pituitary gland 23, 66, 111, 163, 167, 170
plant enzymes 6, 2, 3, 4, 6, 33, 36, 37, 38, 60, 62, 82, 87, 89, 102, 107, 135, 141, 142, 150, 151, 152, 153, 154, 158, 160, 166
plasma proteins 23, 60, 78, 110, 172
potassium 79, 83, 118, 119
preconception 7, 103
precursor 107, 119, 165, 166, 172

pregnancy 6, 7, 8, 13, 43, 48, 64, 67, 69, 74, 75, 76, 80, 84, 91, 92, 94, 97, 98, 99, 100, 102, 103, 105, 108, 109, 110, 111, 112, 113, 114, 115, 120, 131, 132, 133, 135, 136, 168, 169, 173
premenstrual syndrome (PMS) 11, 12, 13, 14, 15, 16, 17, 24, 30, 37, 38, 40, 49, 66, 70, 76, 79, 82, 83, 86, 87, 88, 89, 90, 91, 97, 98, 100, 101, 122, 124, 141, 142, 143, 144, 150, 151, 159, 172, 177, 179
prenatal nutrition 104, 105
procreative abilities 43
progesterone 12, 13, 15, 16, 46, 48, 49, 67, 68, 77, 79, 80, 87, 92, 111, 123, 147, 148, 164
prostaglandins 107
protease 31, 33, 34, 36, 37, 39, 40, 81, 82, 85, 86, 96, 139, 154
protein 2, 3, 22, 23, 24, 27, 29, 30, 31, 32, 34, 39, 40, 41, 52, 53, 54, 55, 58, 59, 60, 61, 62, 75, 76, 77, 78, 80, 81, 82, 85, 86, 87, 89, 91, 96, 97, 98, 99, 100, 101, 109, 110, 111, 112, 113, 114, 115, 117, 118, 119, 120, 122, 129, 135, 140, 141, 142, 143, 144, 150, 151, 154, 157, 160, 161, 162, 166, 167, 169, 170, 173
puberty 43, 50, 70, 91
putrefaction 31

Q

R

receptor site 119, 173

reflex arc 119, 120

reflexes 20

reproductive syndromes 79

reproductive system
 47, 55, 56, 73, 166

respiration 25

rite of passage 44, 48, 146

rituals 44

Romeo and Juliet 63

S

seizure disorder 14

selective serotonin reuptake inhibitors (SSRI) 126, 173

Selye, Hans 24, 26, 52, 90, 178

serotonin 59, 77, 118, 119, 126

sexual arousal 23, 130

Shakespeare 63, 90

shingles 19

shoulder blades 38

somatic 138, 139, 141

sperm count 93, 94

spinal cord 18, 19

starches 96, 164

stimulant 12, 48, 79

stomach acid 32, 75, 82, 87, 88, 89, 99, 101, 109, 110, 122, 140, 168

stress 18, 20, 21, 24, 25, 26, 29, 34, 38, 39, 45, 49, 50, 51, 52, 53, 54, 55, 56, 63, 64, 65, 71, 72, 73, 83, 84, 86, 87, 88, 89, 90, 93, 94, 95, 115, 118, 119, 120, 140, 141, 156, 161, 167

Stress of Life, The 24, 178

stroke 135

sucrase 86, 174

sugar 14, 22, 58, 83, 84, 85, 86, 88, 100, 101, 112, 114, 117, 118, 120, 142, 161, 164, 169, 170, 174

switchboard 18, 21

sympathetic 53, 54, 83, 118, 119, 165

symptom(s) 1, 2, 5, 6, 7, 8, 11, 12, 13, 14, 15, 16, 17, 20, 25, 26, 27, 28, 29, 30, 32, 34, 37, 38, 39, 40, 41, 45, 54, 57, 60, 61, 66, 71, 72, 75, 77, 79, 81, 83, 84, 85, 86, 88, 89, 90, 91, 97, 101, 102, 115, 117, 118, 119, 121, 122, 123, 124, 125, 127, 129, 130, 132, 133, 137, 138, 140, 141, 142, 143, 144, 146, 147, 148, 150, 151, 154, 159, 160, 161, 162, 166, 168, 172, 177

syncope 14

T

testosterone 65, 69

thoracic kyphosis 148

thyroid 1, 23, 54, 87, 111, 112, 126, 168, 174

thyroxine 54, 77, 112

Type A 81, 82, 83, 84

U

Universal Intelligence 21, 24

upper respiratory tract 18

urinalysis 27, 33, 34, 81

uterus 13, 20, 38, 67, 68, 69, 76, 95, 111, 113, 114, 132, 165, 167, 168, 169, 170

V

vagina 67, 148

vegetarian 61, 81, 116

vertigo 14, 125

visceral 18, 19, 20, 26, 27, 30, 37, 90, 138, 139, 140, 142, 174

vitamin 1, 28, 29, 30, 33, 80, 81, 83, 82, 99, 104, 105, 107, 108, 116, 117, 129, 142, 150, 166, 167, 171

voluntary contractions 20

W

waste removal 22, 25

water retention 16

wheat germ 108

Women's Bodies, Women's Wisdom 47, 178

women's nutrition 41

X

X-rays 25

Y

Z

About the Authors

Howard F. Loomis, Jr., D.C., F.I.A.C.A., is a 1967 graduate of Logan Chiropractic College. Dr. Loomis's interest in nutritional food enzymes began when he had the privilege of working with Edward Howell, M.D., the food enzyme pioneer.

He has taught his system to professional health care practitioners since 1985. As founder and president of the Food Enzyme Institute™, he has forged a remarkable career as an educator, having conducted countless seminars in the United States, Canada, Germany, and New Zealand on the clinical identification of food enzyme deficiencies.

He has extensive background in enzymes and enzyme formulations. He is currently president of his own enzyme company, Enzyme Formulations®, Inc. With his exciting approach to health and wellness, Dr. Loomis is now preparing others to take health care into the next century.

Arnold Mann has been writing about medicine for 30 years. His cover stories for *TIME* and *USA Weekend Magazine* have earned him recognition as one of the nation's leading medical journalists. Mr. Mann served as co-author of Dr. Keith Black's book, *Brain Surgeon: A Doctor's Inspiring Encounters with Mortality and Miracles* (Grand Central Publishing, 2010), which was nominated for an NAACP Image Award (Best Nonfiction Book).

Mr. Mann has also written extensively for publications of the National Institutes of Health. He served as personal writer for the Director of the National Cancer Institute, and he oversaw publication of the Institute's *Annual Progress Report to Congress*.

Made in the USA
San Bernardino, CA
05 August 2016